General preface to series

Student textbooks of medicine seek to present the subject of human diseases and their treatment in a manner that is not only informative, but interesting and readily assimilable. It is also important, in a field where knowledge advances rapidly, that the principles are emphasized rather than details, so that information remains valid for as long as possible.

These factors all favour an approach which concentrates on each disease as a disturbance of normal structure and function. Therapy, in principle, follows logically from a knowledge of the disturbance, though it is in this field that the most rapid changes in information occur.

A disturbance of normal structure without any disturbance of function is not important to the patient except for cosmetic or psychological considerations. Therefore, it is the disturbance in function which should be stressed. Preclinical students must get a firm grasp of physiology in a way that shows them how it is related to disease, while clinical students must be presented with descriptions of disease which stress the basic disturbance of function that is responsible for symptoms and signs. This approach should increase interest, reduce the burden on the student's memory and remain valid despite alterations in the details of treatment, so long as the fundamental physiological concepts remain unchallenged.

In the present Series, the major physiological systems are each covered by a pair of books, one preclinical and one clinical, in which the authors have attempted to meet the requirements discussed above. A particular feature is the provision of cross-references between the two members of a pair of books to facilitate the blending of basic science and clinical expertise that is the goal of this Series.

RNH
MH
KBS

Physiological Principles in Medicine

General Editors

Dr R. N. Hardy
Physiological Laboratory, Cambridge

Professor M. Hobsley
Department of Surgical Studies, The Middlesex Hospital and
The Middlesex Hospital Medical School, London

Professor K. B. Saunders
Department of Medicine, St George's Hospital and
St George's Hospital Medical School, London

Respiratory Disorders

Physiological Principles in Medicine

Books are published in linked pairs—the preclinical volume linked to its clinical counterpart, as follows:

Endocrine Physiology by Richard N. Hardy
Clinical Endocrinology by Peter Daggett

Digestive System Physiology by Paul A. Sanford
Disorders of the Digestive System by Michael Hobsley

Respiratory Physiology by John Widdicombe and Andrew Davies
Respiratory Disorders by Ian R. Cameron and Nigel T. Bateman

In preparation:

Neurophysiology by R. H. S. Carpenter
Clinical Neurology by C. D. Marsden

Respiratory Disorders

Ian R. Cameron DM, FRCP

Professor of Medicine, St Thomas's Hospital Medical School, London
Honorary Consultant Physician, St Thomas' Hospital, London

Nigel T. Bateman BM, BCh, MRCP

Consultant Physician, St Thomas' Hospital, London

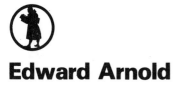

Edward Arnold

First published 1983
by Edward Arnold (Publishers) Ltd.
41 Bedford Square, London WC1B 3DQ

British Library Cataloguing in Publication Data

Cameron, Ian R.
  Respiratory disorders.—(Physiological
  principles in medicine, ISSN 0260-2946)
  1. Respiratory organs—Diseases
  I. Title   II. Bateman, Nigel T.   III. Series
  616.2   RC731
  ISBN 0-7131-4383-5
  ISSN 0260-2946

Filmset in Compugraphic Baskerville by
CK Typesetters Ltd., Sutton, Surrey
and printed in Great Britain by
Thomson Litho Ltd., East Kilbride

Preface

This is a book aimed at medical students. Moreover it is aimed at medical students who wish to read around the subject a little. It is not intended as a terse, fact-filled exam reviser, but to help the student at the transition from basic science to clinical medicine who is wondering how to reconcile the disciplines. He is expected to apply his knowledge of physiology, but it is not obvious how. We hope, therefore, that this brief book will help students, having read the companion book by Widdicombe and Davies, to carry over into clinical medicine the attitudes learnt in basic science. The science of medicine is a delicate flower (the art of medicine is more hardy), and we hope this volume will nurture it.

1983   IRC
                                                                                        NTB

Contents

1

Symptoms and signs of respiratory disease

Introduction

The aim of this book is to relate respiratory diseases and their management to the physiological principles presented in *Respiratory Physiology* by Widdicombe and Davies. In an ideal world, all actions taken in the investigation and treatment of respiratory diseases would be justifiable in terms of basic scientific knowledge. Unfortunately, this is not the case. Sometimes clinicians do things which they know work well but they are unable to explain why. All clinical students must probe their teachers to establish these areas and to determine when the answer 'I don't know' means 'nobody knows but this is what we do'. Respiratory medicine is a specialty in which the basic concepts of physiology are easily applied to disease. For example, an understanding of the mechanisms which control, and the techniques for measuring, airway resistance is important because very common diseases (chronic bronchitis, asthma and emphysema) present as an increased airways resistance. There remain, however, some common disorders in which the basic physiological alterations remain unexplained. This book cannot cover all aspects of respiratory diseases; rather it is an attempt to introduce some of the principles used in classification, diagnosis and treatment.

The first step with any patient will be to take a history and then carry out a careful physical examination. It becomes obvious immediately how difficult it is to relate established clinical methods to basic scientific principles. Some aspects of history taking and examination can only be justified because we know that 'if we do it like this, it works'. In this section attention will be focussed on the aspects of history taking and examination which relate best to our knowledge of structure and function.

Symptoms

Shortness of breath, breathlessness, dyspnoea

One of the commonest symptoms patients present with is described as shortness of breath. The main problem in discussing this symptom is that the term covers a wide variety of sensations which may accompany very different disease processes. Shortness of breath occurs as a symptom of respiratory diseases such as chronic bronchitis, emphysema, asthma and lung fibrosis, but it is also a common feature of heart failure, thyrotoxicosis and anaemia. People also complain of shortness of breath on exercise when they have no disease at all.

Some experts attempt to distinguish two sensations. First, 'shortness of breath': this is the sensation which accompanies an increased ventilation which is essentially normal—that is, the sensation accompanying exercise. If the airways are narrowed (e.g. in asthma), the need for ventilation is made difficult by the increase in airways resistance. This sensation is called 'dyspnoea'. The problem with this division is that it may be clear to the expert but it will not be clear to the patient who will use the terms 'shortness of breath' or 'breathlessness'. We must start from the unsatisfactory position that we use the same term to describe different sensations arising as a consequence of different mechanisms. The experimental situation is just as difficult. Experiments aimed at elucidating these symptoms involve breath-holding, inhaling CO_2 mixtures, breathing hypoxic gas mixtures, breathing against a load (elastic or resistive) and exercise. When interpreting the results of these experiments it is well to remember that they may be investigating different sensations.

There are three sources of evidence that shed some light on the possible mechanism involved:

1. The first experiment examines the view that abnormalities of the arterial Po_2 or Pco_2 are an important determinant of this sensation. Certainly breathing CO_2 or an hypoxic gas mixture gives a sensation of breathlessness, and appropriate manipulation of the Pco_2 or Po_2 before breath-holding will alter the breath-holding time. A key experiment indicates that the breaking point in breath-holding is not determined entirely by Po_2 or Pco_2. If the subject breath-holds to breaking point and then inhales from a bag of gas which will not correct hypoxia or hypercapnia, relief occurs immediately from the sensation of an urgent need for another breath. This occurs without improvement in Pco_2 or Po_2 and suggests that the mechanism forcing a breath at the break-point is not entirely dependent on the level of arterial Po_2 or Pco_2.

2. The view has been advanced that increased afferent nerve impulses from pulmonary receptors are responsible for the sensation of breathlessness. The main supporting evidence comes from experiments with vagal blockade. Blockade of one vagus in normal subjects reduces the ventilatory response to hypercapnia and hypoxia and removes the sensation of breathlessness; breath-holding time is prolonged. In some diseases characterized by severe breathlessness (emphysema, infiltration of the lung), relief can be obtained by the blockade of one vagus. All this certainly suggests that sometimes shortness of breath may be determined by afferent discharges from lung receptors.

3. Another theory suggests that there is a relationship between the ventilatory drive, or the output from the central controlling mechanism, and the ventilation achieved. If this relationship is altered by mechanical distortion (of the airways or chest wall), it may be perceived as shortness of breath. It was predicted that the detection of this inappropriateness depended on muscle contraction; without this, the sensation of shortness of breath should be

abolished. A complicated study showed that the use of curare to paralyse subjects abolished the sensation of breathlessness during breath-holding (i.e. when the paralysed subjects were not ventilated artificially and could not breathe for themselves, they had no sensation of breathlessness). This finding is difficult to interpret. Certainly in this experiment paralysis of the respiratory muscles abolished the sensation, yet in disease states muscle weakness produces a sensation of breathlessness. There is no complete explanation for the origin of this symptom. In all probability there is more than one sensation and these arise because different mechanisms are involved.

When a patient is questioned about shortness of breath, it is essential to try to gauge the impact it has on his life. What does it stop him doing, can he go for walks, play games or run? Has it reduced him to a sedentary life or cost him his job? Sometimes shortness of breath will occur at characteristic times; shortness of breath occurring suddenly at night is typical both of left ventricular failure (when it is called paroxysmal nocturnal dyspnoea) and of asthma.

Cough

This is, again, an extremely common symptom. Coughing occurs because afferent impulses from cough receptors pass up the vagus and initiate the cough. Coughing is brought about by an inspiration followed by an expiration initially against a closed glottis. There is a rise in intrathoracic pressure. When the glottis opens, gas flow through the airways reaches a high velocity; this will tend to clear the airways of sputum or foreign bodies.

Coughing is stimulated by the presence of foreign bodies, excess sputum, irritant gases and closure of airways. If the patient cannot cough adequately then he is unable to clear his airways; this is a serious condition. Failure of the cough mechanism can be caused by muscle weakness or loss of an adequate volume of gas for effective coughing, increased airways resistance limiting gas flow, and paralysis of the vocal cords and laryngeal muscles. Coughing is a characteristic symptom of chronic bronchitis, bronchiectasis, allergic lung diseases, tuberculosis and lung cancer.

Sputum

Sputum production is always abnormal, and examination of the sputum can be important (and easily forgotten). The amount of sputum usually secreted by the bronchial mucosa is swallowed and does not cause a cough. The production of sputum by the goblet cells in the bronchial mucosa constitutes one of the defence mechanisms of the lungs (see Chapter 7). The mucoid sputum is moved towards the mouth by the action of the cilia. On examination, the sputum may have one of several appearances:

1. *White.* This is mucoid sputum; excessive production is a diagnostic feature of chronic bronchitis. In city dwellers there will often be black particles in the sputum.

2. *Thick and sticky, coloured yellow or green.* Generally, sputum with this appearance is caused by infection and the sputum is full of polymorphs when examined microscopically. Purulent sputum is seen in an infective exacerbation in chronic bronchitics, in pneumonia and in bronchiectasis. In patients suffering from bronchiectasis the sputum may be particularly copious and foul-smelling. Not all yellow sputum indicates infection. Sometimes the sputum may be yellow because it is full of eosinophils. This may indicate an allergic process in the lung.

3. *Sometimes the sputum is blood-stained.* Coughing up blood (haemoptysis) is a symptom which must be taken seriously and warrants further investigation. Haemoptysis may vary from the reddish-brown colour sometimes seen in the sputum in pneumonia to frank clots of blood (which may be seen with pulmonary emboli and infarction). Haemoptysis can be a presenting symptom of tuberculosis or lung cancer. In spite of these important causes, many cases of haemoptysis (about 40 per cent) cannot be explained on initial investigation.

Chest pain

The differential diagnosis of chest pain is an enormous subject. Usually in chest medicine two characteristic pains dominate. The first is associated with an upper respiratory tract infection, cough and sore throat. The pain is a central chest pain, described as 'raw and sore'. The pain is worse on coughing; it is usually caused by tracheitis. The second pain is usually felt at the side of the chest. It is sharp and stabbing, and much worse on inspiration or coughing. The patient describes it as 'catching' him during inspiration. This is a pleural pain, usually caused by inflammation of the two layers of pleura.

Smoking

Although smoking habits are not strictly a symptom, an enquiry into smoking is an important part of the history. Precise answers may be difficult to elicit. The information needed is the amount of smoking material the patient has been exposed to. Questions will include the age at which smoking started, the number of cigarettes smoked per day and their tar content. Patients will often claim to have stopped smoking but a few questions will reveal that this was only a few weeks ago when they started to feel ill.

During the history taking there is a good opportunity to observe the patient. Some of the most important observations are the general ones which often are not noted. Maybe this is because they are difficult to quantify, but it is important to note generally whether the patient looks ill, appears to have lost weight, is obviously short of breath or is in pain. Very often in the notes there are many details of specific features of the examination but no general comment on how the patient looked.

Examination

Examination of the respiratory system will usually take place as part of the general examination. Everyone must learn for himself how to put together a scheme for examining patients. This section is about examining the chest; it is not exhaustive but is a critical review of some of the signs which may be elicited.

General features

These fit into any examination, but the following are particularly relevant to the chest.

Cyanosis
This is the blue colour imparted to the skin by the presence of reduced haemoglobin. Because it depends on the absolute amount of reduced haemoglobin present, it is obviously a sign that will occur more readily in a polycythaemic patient than in an anaemic one. Two forms of cyanosis are described:

1. *Central*—the mucous membranes of the mouth and tongue appear blue. This is because something has gone wrong with central gas exchange; the lungs may be diseased or there may be a large right-to-left shunt so that unoxygenated blood reaches the arteries.

2. *Peripheral*—the mucous membranes of the mouth appear pink (normal) but the peripheries (hands and feet) are cold and blue. This implies that there is nothing wrong with gas exchange but that circulatory insufficiency to the limbs has caused a high O_2 extraction from what blood there is. The amount of reduced haemoglobin present is therefore high. This will occur in any condition causing a low cardiac output or intense peripheral vasoconstriction.

Unfortunately, cyanosis is not a very accurate or sensitive physical sign. There will not be agreement among observers on the presence of cyanosis until the Hb saturation has fallen to about 75%.

Enlarged lymph glands
The groups of glands in the neck and axillae are particularly relevant to examination of the chest. Enlarged lymph glands may be very helpful in making the diagnosis (biopsy of a superficial gland is a minor procedure). Discovery of a superficial gland may render a more invasive procedure unnecessary. Enlarged lymph glands may be found in widespread lung cancer, tuberculosis, sarcoid or a lymphoma. In females breast cancer may involve the glands, and the breasts should be examined at the same time.

Clubbing of the fingers
This describes an appearance of the ends of the fingers and the finger nails. It is highly characteristic when fully developed with drumstick ends to the fingers and a nail-bed filled in with spongy, vascular tissue (Fig. 1.1). We have no

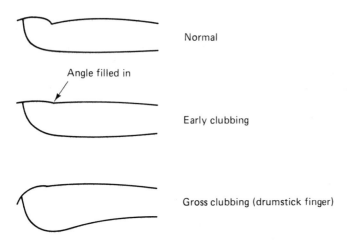

Fig. 1.1 Clubbing of the fingers.

idea what causes clubbing except that there is an increase in local blood flow in the fingers. The importance of this finding lies in its association with various serious diseases, particularly lung cancer, lung abscess, tuberculosis and bronchiectasis. It can also be found with diseases outside the respiratory system; for example, subacute infective endocarditis, primary biliary cirrhosis and ulcerative colitis. Finger clubbing is a good example of pragmatic medicine. It can be an important clue to the presence of a serious disease but it cannot be related to any scientific basis of medicine. It is well to remember that occasionally clubbing is an innocent sign and has been present since birth (congenital clubbing).

Examination of the chest itself

The time-honoured system of clinical examination involves the following steps: inspection, palpation, percussion and auscultation. Each of these methods can be usefully applied to the chest.

Inspection
A long careful look at the chest can elicit a lot of information.

Rate and rhythm of breathing   Is the patient obviously overbreathing? (Under-breathing will not be noticeable.) Is the respiratory rhythm regular and, if not, how is it varying? Cyclical periods of hyperpnoea and hypopnoea are called Cheyne–Stokes breathing. If there is such a periodicity of breathing, a cycle should be timed. Two forms of Cheyne–Stokes breathing occur. One has a long cycle (> 45 seconds), which is usually associated with a prolonged circulation time between the lungs and the chemoreceptors. The control system cannot work properly with such a delay and the system is hunting (which means varying around its desired level). Long-cycle Cheyne–Stokes breathing occurs in severe left ventricular failure. In such cases the cycle can be as long as 2 minutes. This can be produced experimentally in an animal by the introduction of a delay coil into the carotid arteries.

A second form of Cheyne–Stokes breathing occurs with a short cycle (< 45 seconds). This is associated with depression of the central control mechanisms and occurs in some forms of respiratory failure, drug overdose or even, occasionally, in sleep.

Chest shape and respiratory movements   The most important feature is whether the chest is symmetrical and whether the movements are equal on either side. Unequal movements are due to diminished movement on one side and this will usually be the diseased side of the chest wall or lungs.

The chest itself may appear distended, appearing in end-expiration as though the patient had taken a breath in. This is sometimes referred to as a barrel-shaped chest. It is associated with an increased volume of the lungs, which may occur in emphysema or in severe asthma. If the volume of the lungs is increased, the diaphragm will be pushed down and flattened. When the diaphragm contracts in inspiration, instead of pulling upwards and outwards on the ribs, it will pull directly inwards. This pulls the lower ribs in during inspiration instead of out.

If the bellows mechanism of the respiratory pump is working well, equal movements are seen in inspiration. If a segment of the chest wall is unsupported (due to fractured ribs), it will move in during inspiration instead of out, drawn in by the negative intrathoracic pressure. If the airways are narrowed, large negative intrathoracic pressure swings may be generated in inspiration. This will cause the intercostal spaces to be drawn in, indicating the presence of airways obstruction.

Lumps and other abnormal surface features   Do not be led into looking for detail and missing the obvious. Severe distortion of the chest wall and rib cage may lead eventually to respiratory abnormalities. Observe if the spine is twisted (scoliosis) or arched to the front (kyphosis). Obvious lumps or swellings may be seen which will be of importance in interpreting other findings.

Palpation
This will reinforce some of the information gathered by inspection. Placing your hands on the chest will enable you to feel if the movements are equal or not. Any lumps noted can be felt to determine whether they are soft or hard and if they are tender. Any localized tenderness over the ribs can be defined; this may indicate the site of a fracture or some other rib abnormality. One of the most useful things to feel is the position of the trachea. This is felt for in the notch at the top of the manubrium of the sternum. If it is central then the mediastinum is central; alternatively, it may be deviated to the left or the right. If the mediastinal structures are deviated, the reasons for this will have to be ascertained.

Percussion

This is something doctors always do to the chest. Basically, it concerns tapping the chest and noting the noise this makes. Tapping a solid object (e.g. a piece of wood) makes a different noise compared to tapping an air-filled cushion. The chest is described as being resonant on percussion (sounds hollow, this is the normal), hyper-resonant or dull (like the sound over a solid).

1. *Resonant.* This is the usual note and it is detected over normal lungs.

2. *Hyper-resonant.* This is difficult to distinguish from the normal resonant note. Increased 'hollowness' will occur with distended lungs (typically emphysema) or a chest filled with air because the lungs have collapsed (i.e. a pneumothorax).

3. *Dull.* This note is obtained when the lung is solid. This is caused if the lung is airless because it is infiltrated by tumour or full of pneumonic consolidation. A dull note on percussion is also detected when the pleural space is full of fluid (a pleural effusion). Books often mention an area of cardiac dullness but in real life the sign is of little use. An area of dullness may be found anteriorly at the base of the right lung over the liver.

Auscultation

The information gathered by inspection, palpation and percussion is fairly crude. Listening over the lung with a stethoscope produces information which can be more clearly analysed. The noises heard comprise breath sounds and, in some cases, abnormal added sounds.

Breath sounds   When a stethoscope is placed on the chest wall, sounds can be detected accompanying inspiration and expiration. The aim of auscultation is to detect these sounds and, if they are not normal, to make deductions concerning the nature of the disease which has altered them.

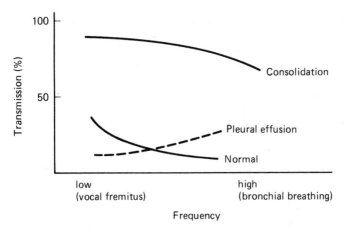

Fig. 1.2 Transmission of sounds through the lungs and chest wall (adapted from Buller & Dornhorst, 1956).

Breath sounds are generated by turbulent air flow in the large airways (the large bronchi). If breath sounds are recorded at the mouth, where they are relatively undistorted by passage through lung tissue, there is a distribution of frequencies between 200 and 2000 Hz. If, on the other hand, they are recorded with a microphone on the chest wall, the frequency range is reduced to 200–600 Hz; in the transmission through the lung tissue most of the high frequencies have been lost.

Changes in the nature of the lung tissue or of other tissues interposed between the generation of the sounds and the listening stethoscope will alter the transmission of these sounds. These changes in the breath sounds can be recognized and associated with the appropriate pathological process. The scientific basis of this is shown in Fig. 1.2. In this diagram the transmission of breath sounds to the chest wall is compared in the normal lung, in the presence of fluid in the pleural space (pleural effusion) and in a lung made solid (consolidation due to pneumonia). The generated sound can be obtained by recording at the mouth or by generating a sound of known frequency; the transmitted sound is then recorded from the chest wall.

Normal lung Low frequencies are transmitted but the higher frequencies are filtered out; this explains the difference between the range of frequencies heard at the mouth and those over the chest wall. High-pitched noises will not be heard through a stethoscope on the chest wall. If you listen with a stethoscope over the larynx, loud, harsh, high-pitched noises accompany inspiration and expiration whereas the breath sounds heard over the chest wall are quieter and of a lower pitch. A high-pitched noise like a whisper is not transmitted through the lung (traditionally the patient is asked to whisper 'twenty-two' in a quiet high-pitched whisper), nor can normal speech be appreciated.

Consolidation A lung which is made solid by consolidation transmits both low and high pitches better than normal lung (see Fig. 1.2). The increased transmission of the high pitches is the easier change to appreciate. This change in transmission is manifest as physical signs which are 'classics' of the chest examination:

1. *Bronchial breathing.* The breath sounds accompanying inspiration and expiration have changed. They are louder and higher pitched; in changing they have become similar to the noises heard over the larynx.
2. *Whispering pectoriloquy.* If the patient whispers a high-pitched quiet 'twenty-two', it can be heard quite clearly with the stethoscope, coming through the abnormal lung.
3. *Aegophony.* Speech sounds come through the chest also, but they are altered in transmission. The transmitted speech has a high-pitched nasal quality (like the bleating of a goat).

Pleural effusion The cut-off in transmission occurs in the low frequencies in the presence of a pleural effusion. If an effusion is very large, no sound will be transmitted at all. With a smaller effusion the sounds which are transmitted will be high-pitched, so bronchial breathing, whispering pectoriloquy and aegophony may be present. The distinction between consolidation and an effusion is made by noting a difference in the transmission of low frequencies. This is best done by making the patient say 'ninety-nine' in a deep gruff voice; that is, he is asked to generate a low-pitched noise. The transmission of low-pitched sound can be detected by listening with the stethoscope; this is called vocal resonance, and it is decreased over a pleural effusion. Alternatively, the same information can be obtained by feeling the chest wall with the palm of a hand (vocal fremitus). Over normal lung the 'thrill' accompanying a deep 'ninety-nine' can be felt. It will be absent over a pleural effusion. It will now be appreciated that patterns of abnormal findings accompany different conditions (Table 1.1).

Table 1.1 Interpretation of physical signs, normal lung, consolidation and pleural effusion

	Findings (on affected side)			
	Movements	Percussion	Breath sounds	Vocal fremitus/ vocal resonance
Normal	Equal	Resonant	Normal	Present
Consolidation	Reduced	Dull	Bronchial breathing	Present
Pleural effusion	Reduced	Dull	Absent or bronchial breathing	Reduced or absent

Added sounds   So far, changes in the transmission of the breath sounds have been described. Finally, it is important to listen for added sounds. The commonest of these are wheezes and crackles.

Wheezes are musical sounds generated during inspiration and expiration. The implication of a wheeze is that airways are narrowed. The exact mechanism which generates a wheeze is not known directly, but there is some indirect evidence which indicates the probable mechanism. Wheezes in the chest do not vary in pitch when the inspired gas is changed from air to a mixture of 80% helium and 20% oxygen (a much less dense mixture). This is surprising because the note of most wind instruments will vary if the density of the gas blowing them is changed. This implies that the wheeze is not generated by a mechanism in which the speed of the sound waves down a pipe is involved (density would change this, making the pitch higher). The length of the pipe will similarly alter the pitch of a wind instrument. A wheeze may alter pitch markedly between inspiration and expiration, which would lead one to suppose that the length of the airway was not important (assuming the wheeze is arising from the same site in expiration and inspiration). Probably a wheeze is generated by an airway whose walls are brought close together, so that they are almost in contact. During gas flow the walls oscillate and the nature of the wheeze depends on the mass and elasticity of the tissues which are oscillating. This mechanism would be expected to be independent of airway length or gas density.

Wheezes are described as monophonic when there is a single source on one pitch; more usually, when they originate from several places, they are polyphonic. Wheezes are commonly heard in all the diseases characterized by airway narrowing, particularly chronic bronchitis, emphysema and asthma.

Crackles are sounds very different from wheezes. They are short, staccato noises rather like a 'popping'. Originally they were taken to imply the presence of fluid in the airways. Clinical and experimental observation, however, does not back this up. Crackles are highly characteristic of some conditions, such as fibrosing alveolitis, where fluid in the airways is not a feature. The best hypothesis available is that a crackle is produced when a small airway opens and there is an explosive change in gas pressure. Crackles can be timed, so they can be described as early or late in inspiration. Sometimes they are present also in expiration (the airway may be opening and closing intermittently depending on local pressure gradients).

Crackles are characteristic of fibrosing alveolitis, especially when they occur late in inspiration; they are also common in pulmonary oedema, pneumonia and chronic bronchitis.

Pleural rub is the other added sound which may be heard; it is due to pleural disease. When heard over the chest, it implies inflammation of the pleural layers. The sound varies, sometimes being a creak and sometimes sounding very like crackles. Pleural rubs can be very short-lived and can vary even from hour to hour. Such a rub will often accompany pleural pain and may be present in pneumonia when the pleura is involved, and sometimes it may occur with a pulmonary embolus or with neoplastic infiltration of the pleura.

At the end of the history taking and examination you should have a firm idea of the problem the patient has and some of the likely causes.

2

Basics of lung disease. Pulmonary function testing

At the simplest level, lung function can be divided into two basic processes. First, the air must be moved into the lungs to reach the gas-exchanging surface, and second, having arrived at this surface, gas exchange between alveolar air and pulmonary capillary blood must proceed so that the blood is oxygenated and carbon dioxide removed. The movement of air into the lungs occurs as a consequence of tidal breathing and requires a conducting system of tubes to reach the gas-exchanging surface. The conducting system comprises the trachea, bronchi, bronchioles and respiratory bronchioles. The gas-exchanging surface occurs in the alveoli at the alveolar/capillary membrane. At this simple level of structure and function, two basic functions—ventilation and gas exchange—can be distinguished, and two associated structures— namely, the airways and the alveoli. Because function and structure are closely related, it is predictable that diseases involving the lung can affect either, or sometimes both, of these processes. There will be, therefore, diseases which affect airways and diseases affecting alveolar tissue, the former leading to defects of ventilation and the latter compromising gas exchange. It is possible to consider the lung, for our purposes, as consisting almost entirely of these two tissues; that is, airways which are supported by the lung parenchyma. Lung parenchyma consists to a large extent of alveolar tissue; alveolar diseases will, therefore, not only affect gas exchange, but also, because of the mechanical and supportive role of lung parenchyma, distort lung mechanics. Throughout this book lung diseases and altered physiology are related to the basic classification shown in Table 2.1.

Table 2.1   Basic classification

Tissue involved	Altered physiology
Airways	Changes in airway resistance
	Abnormal distribution of ventilation in lung
	Abnormalities of total ventilation
Alveolar tissue	Disorders of gas exchange
	Distortion of mechanical properties of lung parenchyma

Inevitably such a simple classification into *airways disease* and *alveolar disease* will have to be elaborated. Some diseases may involve both tissues; for example, emphysema (see Chapter 3) primarily destroys alveolar tissue and thereby reduces the support of the airways, allowing them to collapse. In this classification this is easy to deal with, as emphysema will be described as a primary alveolar, secondary airways disease. Involvement of either system tends to produce a set of physiological abnormalities which are characteristic and a clinical presentation which is quite easily recognized. It is important to realize that this classification can be applied only to generalized disorders of the lung producing defects which are widely distributed. Localized disease may produce regional abnormalities of lung function but these may not be apparent when the common clinical tests of total lung function are used. Certain features of airways and alveolar structure are important in determining their function.

Structure of the airways system

The airways conducting system starts at the mouth and ends in the alveoli. One method of describing this system uses the term 'generations of airways'.

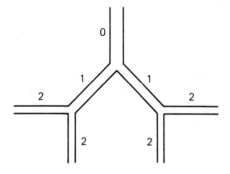

Fig. 2.1 Airways pattern and its description in 'generations'. The trachea is generation 0, the main bronchi are generation 1, and so on, the divisions reaching generation 23.

In this system the trachea is generation 0, the right and left main bronchi generation 1, and so on (Fig. 2.1). Twenty-three generations of airways are described and these may be broadly divided into those which are purely conductive, some which are purely concerned with gas exchange and an intermediate zone (Table 2.2).

Each airway when it divides gives rise to a pair of daughter airways, each having a diameter slightly less than that of the parent airway. Although at each division airways themselves become smaller, the total cross-sectional area of the airways will increase (Fig. 2.2). The air inspired will all pass through the trachea, but this volume will have been subdivided many times before the alveoli are reached. This has important implications for the distribution of

Table 2.2   Generations of airways

Generation	Function
0–16	Purely conductive
17–19	Transition – respiratory bronchioles. Conductive with some respiratory tissue
20–23	Respiratory. Alveolar ducts and sacs

resistance to gas flow between the large (central) airways and the smaller (peripheral) airways. Instinctively one would predict that the maximum site of resistance to gas flow would occur in the small (peripheral) airways. More detailed consideration reveals that this is not so. If, at each airway division, gas flow is halved yet the total cross-sectional area increases, clearly for a given flow the greatest cross-sectional area occurs at the periphery and the smallest centrally (Fig. 2.2). The major site of resistance to air flow will occur in the large, central airways. Many techniques have been devised for dividing the resistance of the entire conducting system into a proportion due to the large, central airways and a proportion due to the smaller, peripheral airways. There will also be a contribution to the total resistance from the larynx and pharynx (Table 2.3).

The important fact to be retained from these observations is that when we measure, or use an indirect method to assess, the resistance of all the airways together, the result will be largely determined by events in the larger, more central airways. Changes in the resistance of the peripheral airways will contribute proportionally so little that they will be lost in the total measurement. It is for this reason that the peripheral airways have been called the 'silent zone' of the lung. This would not matter if these airways were unimportant in diseases, but histological evidence indicates that some common airways diseases may start in the small airways. Our hopes of detecting the early effects of these diseases (e.g. the changes due to cigarette smoking) are reduced because the measurements in common usage are

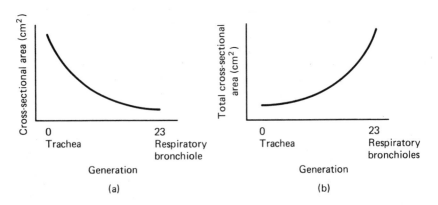

Fig. 2.2   (a) Cross-sectional area of an airway. (b) *Total* cross-sectional area of the airways.

Table 2.3 Contribution of the larynx, pharynx, large airways and small airways to total airways resistance

	kPa · l^{-1} · s^{-1} (cmH$_2$O · l^{-1} · s^{-1})	Percentage of total
Larynx and pharynx	0.05 (0.5) ⎱	84
Large airways (dia. > 2 mm)	0.05 (0.5) ⎰	
Small airways (dia. < 2 mm)	0.02 (0.2)	16

insensitive to events in the small airways. There has been, therefore, a need to devise tests which assess function in this part of the airways system.

The airways system described is one of symmetrically branching tubes; this is suspiciously simple for real life. Detailed investigations have revealed that the branching system is far from symmetrical. Nevertheless, the conclusions reached above are well founded and the implications for the site of, and the measurement of, airways resistance can stand.

Ways in which airways can become narrowed

The various processes which may cause narrowing of the airways are listed below. (The mechanisms concerned and their consequences are considered in more detail in Chapter 3.)

1. Increase in bronchial smooth muscle tone.
2. Swelling of the mucosal membrane due to:
   (a) inflammation;
   (b) oedema;
   (c) enlargement of the mucus-secreting glands.
3. Presence of excess mucus.
4. Loss of support (i.e. lack of tension of tissues on bronchial wall).

The term 'narrowing of the airways' has been used above. Most clinical tests use the term 'airways obstruction' but it has been pointed out that true obstruction does not always occur; for this reason, some people prefer the term 'air-flow limitation'. Throughout this book, however, 'airways obstruction' has been used, as a more graphic term.

Structure and abnormalities of the gas-exchanging tissues

The structure of the tissues concerned with gas exchange are described both in Widdicombe and Davies: *Respiratory Physiology*, Chapter 1 and in Chapter 4 of this book. At this stage it will suffice to indicate that gas exchange depends on the function of the alveoli and the pulmonary capillaries. Lung parenchyma is composed of these structures and the interstitial space of the lung. Diseases of the lung parenchyma may alter the function of these tissues in several ways:

1. By accumulation of fluid in the alveoli and/or the interstitial space of the lung (pulmonary oedema or inflammation, see Chapter 4).

2. By the presence of fibrosis in the alveolar wall or interstitial space, leading to shrinkage and stiffening of the tissues (lung fibrosis, see Chapter 4).

3. By destruction of alveolar tissue, which occurs in emphysema (see Chapter 3). If the alveoli are destroyed (rather than splinted by fibrosis), the lung becomes 'floppy' and the unsupported airways tend to collapse.

These structural changes will lead to defects of gas exchange and an alteration in the mechanical properties of the lungs.

Assessment of pulmonary function

The testing of lung function can be made into a very complicated subject. This is not necessary and very simple tests can be used to obtain most of the information required in making a diagnosis. In this section only very simple tests will be described. Every patient suspected of having respiratory disease should be assessed by spirometry (the only exception to this is the patient suspected of having active tuberculosis: for obvious reasons, he should *not* blow into the spirometer). Spirometry is extremely simple and provides information quickly which is diagnostically valuable.

The spirometer used may be of a variety of types; it may be wet or dry, and the answers may be given as a graph or by digital read-out. Essentially, the spirometer must be capable of giving two pieces of information:

1. The volume which the subject exhales.
2. The time taken to exhale any given volume.

The essential measurement is the volume expired when the subject exhales as much as he can from a maximum inspiration—or, in other words, when he goes from total lung capacity (TLC) to residual volume (RV). The volume exhaled is the vital capacity (VC)—and, because in this case the subject is urged to blow out *as hard and as fast as possible*, it is the forced vital capacity (FVC). Using the timing mechanism of the spirometer, the volume exhaled in one second is also measured; this is the forced expiratory volume in one second (FEV_1). In simple terms, the information obtained is the volume which the subject can blow out and the proportion blown out in the first second.

It is worth considering the defects of this method of assessing lung function. We are assessing pulmonary mechanics under rather an odd situation—that is, when the subject stresses the lungs mechanically by a maximum forced expiration; among other things, this will tend to compress the lungs and, hence, the airways. If the airways are abnormal, perhaps lacking support from diseased parenchyma, this manoeuvre will tend to make them collapse. So, like all systems of measurement, it has its defects and the methodology may affect the findings; that is to say, the results obtained during a forced expiration apply to this situation only, if we are to be rigid. Nevertheless, the technique is extremely useful and enables us to distinguish three patterns observed during a forced exhalation (Fig. 2.3), as follows.

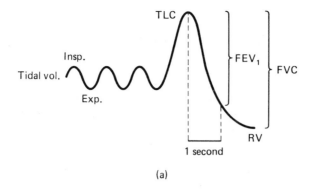

(a)

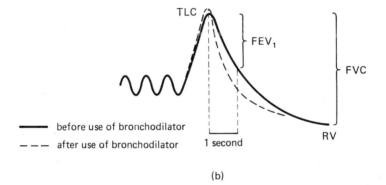

(b)

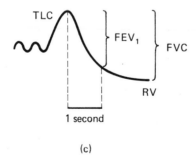

(c)

Fig. 2.3 Spirometry. (a) Normal: $FEV_1/FVC > 80\%$ (example: $4.7/5.1 = 92.2\%$). (b) Obstructive: $FEV_1/FVC < 80\%$ (examples: $2.0/4.0 = 50\%$ before bronchodilatation; $2.9/4.2 = 69\%$ after bronchodilatation). (c) Restrictive: $FEV_1/FVC > 80\%$ (example: $1.8/2.0 = 90\%$; predicted values for this should have been $4.4/5.1$).

Normal

When the subject exhales forcibly from TLC to RV, the FEV_1 and FVC are measured. Two separate pieces of information are obtained from these figures. The first indicates whether the volumes of FEV_1 and FVC are within the range predicted for that individual's size, age and sex (these figures can be obtained from standard tables). Obviously, lung volumes will vary with body size, and an FVC appropriate to a 1.5 m (5 ft) 70-year-old female would not be appropriate in a 1.8 m (6 ft) 20-year-old male. Second, information is derived from the ratio FEV_1/FVC expressed as a percentage. A normal person will be able to blow out 80 per cent or more of the VC in the first second, but this ability may be compromised by airway disease (see below). The normal pattern (Fig. 2.3a) consists, therefore, of lung volumes within the predicted range for that subject and an FEV_1/FVC greater than 80 per cent.

Obstructive

This pattern is seen in airways diseases. The main feature is that the subject takes a long time to exhale his VC, resulting in a reduction in the FEV_1. This reduction may be considerable, and in a patient with severe airways disease the ratio FEV_1/FVC may fall below 50 per cent. The FVC may also be reduced, but this is not a striking feature of the condition. The trace from the spirometer is highly characteristic (Fig. 2.3b).

Once it has been established that the subject has an obstructive pattern on spirometry one further piece of invaluable information can be obtained: can the airways obstruction be reversed? The simplest way of testing this in the clinic, pulmonary function laboratory or at the bedside is by administration of a β_2 stimulant drug (a bronchodilator) as an aerosol. As a general rule, salbutamol is used (100 μg). The forced exhalation is then repeated and any change in the FEV_1/FVC ratio is noted. If the airway disease is reversible by β-stimulation, the ratio will improve; obviously if the disease is irreversible, there is no change. An improvement in the ratio is not the only change which can be seen. Sometimes there will be a greater increase in FVC than in FEV_1, with a consequent reduction in the FEV_1/FVC ratio. The essential feature one is seeking after use of a bronchodilator drug is a change. This gives rise to a question dreaded by respiratory physiologists—how much change respresents a 'significant change' (significant in the functional rather than the statistical sense)? The probable answer is an improvement in the FEV_1/FVC ratio or FEV_1 greater than 15–20 per cent. This is extremely important because it carries implications for diagnosis and, obviously, for treatment. If the airways obstruction can be demonstrated to be *reversible* (i.e. the spirometry changes towards normal after bronchodilatation, dotted line in Fig. 2.3b), then the diagnosis will be asthma (see Chapter 3) and the subject will be well advised to use a bronchodilator spray therapeutically. If, on the other hand, the obstruction is *irreversible*, then the cause is likely to be chronic bronchitis or emphysema.

Restrictive

This pattern is seen when the lung parenchyma is involved with disease causing extensive fibrosis or scarring. Because the fibrous tissue shrinks and is relatively non-elastic, the lungs are small and stiff; if the parenchyma alone is involved, the airways function remains normal. On forced exhalation, therefore, the characteristic finding is a reduction in the FEV_1 and FVC, both of which may be well below the figure predicted for that individual. Because the airways are normal, the proportion of the FVC blown out in the first second will still be 80 per cent or more. An example of this abnormality is given in Fig. 2.3c. This pattern of abnormality is seen in diseases which involve lung parenchyma extensively such as fibrosing alveolitis, sarcoid and the pneumoconioses.

The simple non-invasive manoeuvre of a forced exhalation allows us to recognize these three patterns—normal, obstructive and restrictive. It is worth emphasizing that spirometry will only show abnormalities in generalized lung disease; local disease such as pneumonia or a lung cancer will not influence these findings. In these conditions the diagnostic information is obtained by a different investigative pathway (see Chapters 7 and 10). Like all simple tests, exhalation spirometry depends on certain technical features being satisfied or the results may be meaningless. These are worth considering in detail, as spirometry is often considered such a lowly measurement that it is poorly supervised. It is not unusual for results to be obtained from an instrument which is broken or has never been calibrated. Incorrect results once recorded in the patient's notes may be a greater hazard than no results at all.

Technical considerations for successful spirometry

1. The spirometer itself must be adequate. Spirometers should be, although all too often they are not, regularly calibrated. Instruments which are obviously unsatisfactory should never be used. Always suspect and investigate results which go against common sense.

2. The blow must be technically satisfactory; that is, the subject must make an adequate effort, and you can usually judge this. Look carefully for leaks around the mouthpiece and nose, and make sure that the subject does not close his glottis. Most subjects will require, at least the first time, patient coaching.

3. There has been some controversy over the number of trials the patient should have. The recommendation of the Medical Research Council is to take three technically satisfactory exhalations after two practice attempts. The mean of the three test blows should then be used.

4. It is worth recording the time of day as well as the date. Lung function may vary from day to day and in asthmatics there may be a pronounced diurnal variation.

5. The results must be corrected to body temperature and pressure, saturated (BTPS).

6. The use of a bronchodilator to establish the presence or absence of reversibility must be adequately supervised. Two common errors frequently arise. First, the spray is used incorrectly as it is extremely difficult to inhale the full dose. Obviously, if this is not done properly there will be a reduced effect. Most subjects require practice, and dummy sprays are available for this. Second, after the spray has been used successfully it is essential to wait long enough before repeating the spirometry (5–20 minutes depending on the bronchodilator used). All too often this is done immediately and a false verdict of irreversible obstruction may be recorded.

Correctly performed spirometry allows us to diagnose with confidence either an obstructive or a restrictive defect suggesting either an abnormality of the airways or the lung parenchyma (remember that this is largely composed of alveolar tissue).

Measurement and interpretation of arterial blood gas tensions

The other basic information, essential in the testing of lung function, is the measurement of the arterial blood gas tensions (Pa_{CO_2} and Pa_{O_2}). This requires an arterial puncture, so that it is invasive. The technique for arterial puncture is not best described in a book, but with care and patience it should be painless and there should not be a painful haematoma afterwards.

The importance of the measurement of blood gas tensions lies in the fact that it represents a final assessment of the effectiveness of breathing. Remember that breathing is required to oxygenate arterial blood and remove carbon dioxide. The effectiveness of the two basic processes—ventilation and gas exchange—is assessed by these measurements. It is possible to set limits on the arterial gas tensions and to define levels of abnormality which indicate *respiratory failure* (see Chapter 5).

The sample of arterial blood must be taken anaerobically. If there is to be a delay of more than 10 minutes before the measurements are made, the syringe should be stored in ice. The P_{O_2}, P_{CO_2} and pH of the sample are measured in appropriate electrodes. These are now made for routine use and are relatively simple to use, and, as with so much equipment, almost anyone can obtain *some* answer. Obtaining accurate measurements routinely is a matter of some skill. On any occasion when there is a gross discrepancy in the results or an extraordinary answer, *always* check for a technical error. The electrodes require careful maintenance and calibration, and, like all equipment, they can, and do, go wrong. It is usually said that the 'normal' arterial blood gas tensions are a P_{O_2} of 12 kPa (90 mmHg), a P_{CO_2} of 5.3 kPa (40 mmHg) (with a range of 4.7–6 kPa or 35–45 mmHg) and a pH of 7.35–7.45. The Pa_{O_2} varies with age (Fig. 2.4), so in a patient of 80 years a Pa_{O_2} as low as 8–9.3 kPa (60–70 mmHg) may be normal.

Respiratory failure is defined as a Pa_{O_2} below 8 kPa (60 mmHg) and/or a Pa_{CO_2} above 6.5 kPa (49 mmHg). This definition needs qualifying to be precise. The subject must at rest, at sea level and breathing ambient air. Using this definition of respiratory failure, two patterns of arterial blood gas tensions can be discerned:

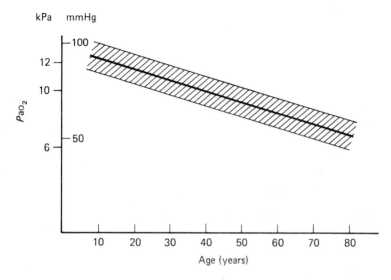

Fig. 2.4 Variation of arterial Po_2 with age (shaded area is regression line ± 2 SD).

1. A low Pao_2, below 8 kPa (60 mmHg), and a raised $Paco_2$ above 6.5 kPa (49 mmHg). This is hypoxic, hypercapnic respiratory failure.

2. Again a low Pao_2, but in this group of patients the $Paco_2$ is normal or, more usually, below normal—i.e. 4–4.7 kPa (30–35 mmHg). This is hypoxic, normocapnic or hypocapnic respiratory failure.

These categories are of extreme importance, as they carry implications for diagnosis and treatment (this is considered in more detail in Chapter 5). The importance at this stage lies in the causes of these two distinct patterns, which may be related to the two different types of altered physiology.

Hypoxic, hypercapnic respiratory failure

This section is concerned with the mechanisms responsible for hypoxic, hypercapnic respiratory failure. The causes in terms of disease and appropriate therapy are considered in Chapter 5. It is obvious that if one stops breathing, the Pao_2 must fall and the $Paco_2$ rise; this pattern of arterial blood gases can come about, therefore, by not breathing enough. This is called *alveolar hypoventilation*. The effect of changes in the level of ventilation on arterial blood gases is shown in Fig. 2.5. As alveolar ventilation falls, so alveolar and arterial Po_2 fall and Pco_2 increases. Ventilation may be looked upon as the mechanism whereby oxygen is added to, and CO_2 removed from, alveolar air. As is discussed in Chapter 5, there are many lesions which can impair an individual's ability to ventilate. Because we are concerned at the moment with diseases in the lungs, we can limit these possibilities; it is diseases of the airways which give rise to this form of respiratory failure. It is

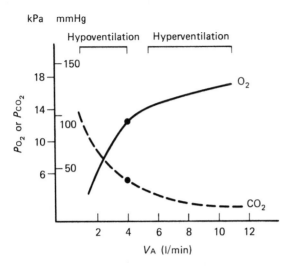

Fig. 2.5   Effect of ventilation on alveolar gas tension.

easy to suppose that severe airways obstruction, which may come about as a consequence of either chronic bronchitis or asthma, may so interfere with the subject's ability to ventilate that eventually he comes to 'tolerate' the low PaO_2 and raised $PaCO_2$. Such a situation in a normal individual would be intolerable, the hypoxic and hypercapnic stimuli unleashing a colossal drive to ventilate. Why do these subjects tolerate this situation? In short, this is not known. The association of this pattern of respiratory failure with airways disease emphasizes the classification given in Table 2.1, lung diseases being divided up according to their impact on airways or alveolar disease. Unfortunately, the two types of respiratory failure cannot be rigidly associated, one with airways disease and the other with alveolar disease. This 'untidiness' is discussed after considering the other type of respiratory failure.

Hypoxic, hypocapnic respiratory failure

This type of respiratory failure occurs as a result of a very different mechanism, and is rather harder to understand. The problem posed is how can the patient become hypoxic while at the same time retaining the ability to hold his $PaCO_2$ below normal? The answer lies in the shape of the oxygen and carbon dioxide dissociation curves (Fig. 2.6), and the fact that the $PaCO_2$ is directly related to the level of ventilation:

$$PaCO_2 = \frac{CO_2 \text{ production}}{\text{ventilation}} \times K$$

where K is a factor to produce the correct units. If CO_2 production remains constant, $PaCO_2$ depends entirely on the level of ventilation. We can state a general rule (very unusual in medicine): 'if the $PaCO_2$ is too high the individual

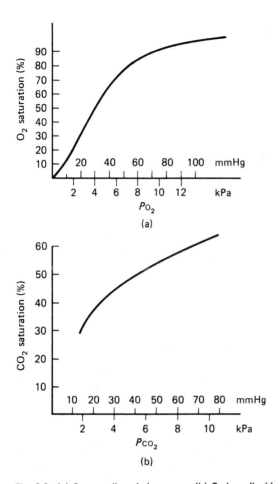

Fig. 2.6 (a) Oxygen dissociation curve. (b) Carbon dioxide dissociation curve.

is ventilating too little, and if the Pa_{CO_2} is low he is ventilating too much; if the Pa_{CO_2} is normal that subject is ventilating an adequate amount for his CO_2 production'. Clearly in the type of respiratory failure we are discussing (with a low or normal Pa_{CO_2}) the patient has retained his ability to ventilate adequately. The explanation for the arterial hypoxaemia must lie in inadequate gas exchange. Understanding the mechanism responsible requires consideration of the consequences of mismatch of ventilation to perfusion in the lung (see Chapter 2; and Widdicombe and Davies: *Respiratory Physiology*, Chapter 6) as well as the shape of the dissociation curves. In order to revise the consequences of ventilation/perfusion mismatching, look at Fig. 2.7. In the lung unit shown, total alveolar ventilation is maintained normal (4 litres per minute) and so is pulmonary blood flow (5 litres per minute). A patchily distributed disease has resulted in relatively too much ventilation in alveolus A

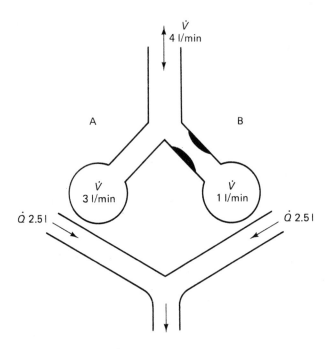

Fig. 2.7   Unevenness of alveolar ventilation. A: $\dot{V}_A/\dot{Q} = 3.0/2.5$. B: $\dot{V}_A/\dot{Q} = 1/2.5$.

(3 litres per minute) for the blood flow (2.5 litres per minute), whereas in alveolus B (ventilation 1 litre per minute, perfusion 2.5 litres per minute) there is too little ventilation for the perfusion (a low $\dot{V}_A/\dot{Q}$ ratio, a contribution to the venous admixture effect; see Widdicombe and Davies: *Respiratory Physiology*, Chapter 6, to revise these terms). Blood coming from the under-ventilated unit B must have a low P_{O_2} and saturation. The question is, can the overventilated alveolus A 'make up' for the poor perfusion of alveolus B and so correct the gas tensions in the mixed blood coming from both of them? If the shape of the oxygen dissociation curve is considered, it is apparent that alveolus A is on the flat part of the curve and cannot therefore compensate for the hypoxic blood leaving alveolus B. In simple terms, blood from a 'good' part of the lung cannot be 'supercharged' with oxygen to make up for a poorly performing area. This is not so for carbon dioxide because the dissociation curve is virtually linear over the range we are considering. Because of this, a region with a high $\dot{V}_A/\dot{Q}$ ratio (alveolus A) can compensate for an alveolus with a low ratio (alveolus B). Because overall arterial hypoxia results, this will continue to drive ventilation and keep P_{aCO_2} at a level below the normal. In this way uneven distribution of ventilation leads to arterial hypoxia and hypocapnia. When this pattern is seen in a patient, we can predict with confidence that the problem is one of inadequate gas exchange and that this has occurred as a result of ventilation/perfusion mismatch. It is worth making clear at this point that it is the unevenness of ventilation and perfusion which

causes the trouble. A total reduction in ventilation must result in hypercapnia as well as hypoxia; in the example shown above, impaired gas exchange produces hypoxia but the patient has retained the ability to control his $P\text{aco}_2$.

As indicated earlier, the classification into obstructive and restrictive defects from the results of spirometry and two sorts of respiratory failure from the arterial gases is not totally 'tidy'. To make life simple, airways disease should lead to hypoxic, hypercapnic respiratory failure and alveolar disease to hypoxic hypocapnia. This is predictably not so. As emphasized, the maldistribution of ventilation, which occurs because diseases are not symmetrical in their involvement of airways, sometimes leads to hypoxia and hypocapnia in airway disease. This spoils our classification; in asthma, for example, which is entirely an airways disease, either type of respiratory failure can occur. In general it is the more severe asthmatic who ceases to ventilate adequately (developing a raised $P\text{aco}_2$) whereas the less severe asthma attack produces hypoxia with a reduced $P\text{aco}_2$.

It is necessary to take this a step further because the two mechanisms leading to respiratory failure can coexist. Clearly, patients with airways disease sufficiently severe to lead to hypercapnic, hypoxic respiratory failure will also have sufficient airways disease to have an underlying ventilation/perfusion defect. The group of patients who develop hypercapnia are unable, for unknown reasons, to remedy the situation by hyperventilation. Finally, we can make our best classification of disordered lung function as shown in Table 2.4.

Table 2.4 Correlation of pathological lesion, physiological abnormalities and disease

Pathological lesion	Spirometry	Arterial gases	Disease
Primary airways disease	Obstructive	Uneven distribution of ventilation $\downarrow Po_2$ $\downarrow Pco_2$	Asthma Chronic bronchitis
		Alveolar hypoventilation $\downarrow Po_2$ $\uparrow Pco_2$	
Primary alveolar disease	Restrictive	Uneven distribution of ventilation and perfusion $\downarrow Po_2$ $\downarrow Pco_2$	Fibrosing alveolitis Sarcoid
Mixed (i.e. primary alveolar, secondary airway)	Obstructive	Uneven distribution of ventilation and perfusion $\downarrow Po_2$ $\downarrow Pco_2$	Emphysema

In order to achieve this simple classification only the results of spirometry and blood gas tension measurements have been used. Further tests of lung function may give additional, useful information. One of the most useful, and certainly the simplest is the measurement of the peak expiratory flow rate.

Peak expiratory flow rate

This is one of the most convenient and widely used tests of respiratory function. Like all tests it has its advantages and disadvantages, but once these

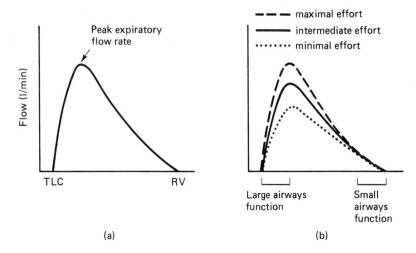

Fig. 2.8 Flow during a forced exhalation from TLC to RV (flow/volume curve). (a) Flow/volume relation during forced exhalation. (b) Effect of effort on the manoeuvre.

have been recognized it can be very valuable. The measurement requires an instrument which will record the highest flow rate achieved during a maximum expiratory effort. Many of the comments relevant to forced exhalation spirometry apply again. Figure 2.8 shows exactly what happens to expiratory flow rate as the subject forcibly exhales from high lung volume (TLC) down to RV. The peak expiratory flow rate (PEFR) is only one piece of information which can be gained from this manoeuvre. Most of the instruments used record only the PEFR. The most widely used of these is the Wright peak flow meter (this relies on the deflection of a vane) although there are now cheaper instruments (the peak flow gauge) available and some which are even disposable. If the complete exhalation is recorded on an *x–y* recorder so that one can see flow rates at all lung volumes (Fig. 2.8a), it becomes obvious that the peak expiratory flow rate is rapidly achieved at high lung volumes. Flow rate falls off as RV is approached. In Fig. 2.8b the effect of varying the expiratory effort is shown. Unfortunately, PEFR is highly effort-dependent. It is up to the observer to obtain a maximum effort from the subject and to see that the test is correctly performed. It is also obvious in Fig. 2.8b that although the *peak* expiratory flow rate is highly effort-dependent, flow rates at low lung volumes are not. They are likely, therefore, to be more reproducible. In addition, there are good reasons for thinking that the expiratory flow rate at low lung volumes depends on the air flow in the small (peripheral) airways whereas at high lung volumes (where PEFR occurs) flow depends on the function of the larger (central) airways. There are advantages to be gained by recording flow rates at low lung volumes, and this is becoming a more frequent measurement as the quest continues for a test to assess small airways function. The effort dependency of the PEFR is an obvious disadvantage.

The PEFR is a complex measurement although it is very simple to perform. The highest flow rate achieved depends first on airways function (i.e. air flow in the large central airways) but it will also be influenced by the elastic recoil of the lung. Inhaling to TLC stretches the lung parenchyma and when the subject 'lets go' to exhale forcibly, the elastic recoil of the lung will contribute to the driving force. Elastic recoil is a function of the 'stretchiness' or compliance of the lung parenchyma which will be altered in diseases which affect this tissue; these are, of course, the diseases of alveolar tissue. The conclusion is that PEFR can be reduced below the predicted level by diseases of the airways and of alveolar tissue. Because the PEFR is effort-dependent, it can obviously be reduced by any disease which impairs the function of the respiratory muscles or their ability to move the rib cage. It is not a specific measurement of any particular physiological function. Reduction of the PEFR indicates 'something wrong with the respiratory system' in a broad sense but does not tell us what. It may be likened to a 'sort of respiratory ESR'. This feature is one of the strengths and one of the weaknesses of the measurement. It is an advantage if it is being used as a general screening test—e.g. this patient is short of breath, is it due to a respiratory disease? It is also useful to epidemiologists who may require a simple test, easily applicable to large numbers of individuals, to assess any respiratory impairment. It will *not* be useful, as spirometry is, in differentiating one type of respiratory disorder from another.

Once a more precise diagnosis has been made, the PEFR is an excellent measurement for assessing variation of the disease or the effect of treatment because it is so easy to perform at the bedside (in hospital or at home) or in the clinic. This is particularly useful when information is required regarding variation of a disease with time. This occurs with asthmatics who may be extremely well when seen in the clinic yet suffer from severe attacks at night. Lung function tests done in the laboratory in the day time may be normal.

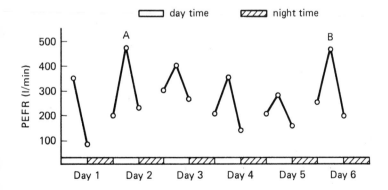

Fig. 2.9 Use of peak expiratory flow rate to show changes in pulmonary function over an extended period. (NB. The measurements made in the clinic at points A and B may be highly unrepresentative.)

The patient can be taught to measure and record his own PEFR, which may reveal, as in Fig. 2.9, that although he was well during the day and during clinic attendance, a severe reduction of lung function occurred at night. This type of information can be extremely useful in diagnosis and in monitoring treatment.

In summary, it might be said that the peak flow meter, although not the prime instrument of the respiratory physiologist, should be as common in a doctor's equipment (be he hospital or community based) as a sphygmomano-meter.

Other, more specialized, tests of lung function

The tests described so far—namely, spirometry (FEV_1 and FVC), arterial blood gas tensions and PEFR—will supply the information necessary in the majority of cases. Under some circumstances more complicated tests may be necessary. In the main, further information may be needed (1) if the clinical situation is complicated or (2) if a major therapeutic decision hinges on the results. As an example of the former, it may be difficult to decide in someone with chronic disease of the heart valves how much of the dyspnoea is due to heart disease and how much due to lung disease. Certainly the decision to replace one or more heart valves is a major therapeutic decision and under these circumstances it may be necessary to make more precise measurements of lung function to back up spirometry. The patient's symptoms, which usually include dyspnoea, will respond poorly to valve replacement if they are due to lung disease.

Measurement of lung volumes

Most pulmonary function laboratories measure lung volumes. The volumes measured are VC, TLC, FRC (functional residual capacity) and RV. In general, these will merely augment the volumes obtained by spirometry. The results may indicate reduced lung volumes, as occurs in the restrictive defects seen with fibrosing alveolitis and other conditions causing small scarred lungs. On the other hand, lungs affected by emphysema may show increased lung volumes. When there is severe airways obstruction as in status asthmaticus, there may be air-trapping leading to hyperinflated lungs and increased lung volumes.

Transfer factor

Often very useful clinically, this is a measure of the ability of the lungs to transfer gas from alveolar air to the blood. The most common method in use measures the transfer of carbon monoxide, which has a molecular weight close to that of oxygen and also combines with haemoglobin. It is, of course, used in very low concentration (0.3% in the inspired gas mixture). The usual method (the single-breath method) requires that the subject can hold his breath for at least 10 seconds and expire a volume in excess of 1 litre (this is often not possible in patients with a severe restrictive defect). The amount of carbon monoxide which is transferred out of alveolar air is calculated from:

1. The difference in concentration between the inspired and the expired carbon monoxide. This fall in concentration during the 10-second breath-hold depends on the movement of carbon monoxide out of alveolar air into blood and the initial dilution which occurs when the gas containing carbon monoxide is inhaled. The dilution which occurs will depend on the volume of gas in the alveoli and airways at that time. This can be corrected for as described below.

2. Measuring the dilution of an inert gas such as helium. Helium will not be absorbed from alveolar air because it is so insoluble, and the fall in helium concentration between inspired and expired air will depend solely on dilution by the gas already present in the lung. This will indicate what proportion of the fall in carbon monoxide concentration can be attributed to dilution and how much to transfer into blood. Transfer factor is measured in units of $mmol \cdot min^{-1} \cdot kPa^{-1}$ ($ml \cdot min^{-1} \cdot mmHg^{-1}$).

This test is particularly sensitive to damage of alveolar tissue, with loss of area for gas exchange. It will often be strikingly abnormal before lung mechanics or arterial blood gas tensions have changed. It is primarily used in the diagnosis of diseases such as sarcoid and fibrosing alveolitis and in monitoring the effect of treatment. It may also be used to help in distinguishing emphysema from asthma and chronic bronchitis. All three diseases produce airways obstruction but only in emphysema is there alveolar damage and consequently a reduction in the transfer factor. It is a useful test because it is easy to perform, quick and non-invasive, and will give early evidence of alveolar damage. When corrected for alveolar volume it is called the transfer coefficient.

Two further measurements of lung function may sometimes be necessary for precise diagnosis. They are also of interest because they represent the definitive measurements for assessing airways disease and parenchymatous disease. They are (1) measurement of airways resistance and (2) measurement of lung compliance.

Airways resistance (R_{aw})

It is beyond the scope of this book to describe the various techniques for measuring airways resistance (R_{aw}) and their problems. The most satisfactory measurement available now is made in the body plethysmograph. This is an airtight box in which the subject must sit while the measurement is made. R_{aw} is measured in units of $kPa \cdot l^{-1} \cdot s^{-1}$ ($cmH_2O \cdot l^{-1} \cdot s^{-1}$). It has the advantage over spirometry that it is a direct measurement of the required variable rather than an indirect assessment.

Compliance

Lung compliance is a measure of the distensibility of the lungs in terms of the amount they will expand when a given pressure is applied. Over a range of inspired volumes the pressure applied to the lung (the transpulmonary pressure) is measured. Compliance is obtained from the relation between volume and transpulmonary pressure in units of l/kPa (l/cmH$_2$O). Although it is the definitive measurement of the 'stiffness' of the lungs, it is seldom required clinically. More often the impact of diseases causing stiff, small lungs is assessed from the lung volumes and the transfer factor.

3

Airways obstruction

In Chapter 2 respiratory disorders were classified into two major groups: diseases of the airways and diseases of alveolar tissue. In this chapter the conditions which cause airways obstruction will be discussed in more detail: chronic bronchitis, emphysema and asthma. These are common diseases and they illustrate between them the different mechanisms which can cause narrowing of the airways.

Mechanisms of airways narrowing

There are relatively few factors which can narrow airways and increase airways resistance:

1. Active constriction of the bronchial smooth muscle.
2. Plugging of the airways by excess production of mucus or by infected mucus.
3. Inflammation of the bronchial mucosa with accompanying swelling.
4. Loss of support for the airways, because of destruction of the surrounding lung, with consequent airways collapse.

The three common diseases which result in airway narrowing—chronic bronchitis, emphysema and asthma—depend on different primary mechanisms in bringing this about. In asthma, airways narrowing is caused by active bronchoconstriction, the essential feature of a simple attack. Certainly in more complicated asthma, mucus plugging or infection may play a part, but active bronchoconstriction is the major component. Chronic bronchitis is characterized by changes in the bronchial mucosa, increased secretion of mucus and repeated infection leading to airways narrowing. Lastly, emphysema—essentially a disease destructive of alveolar tissue—destroys the support of the airways, allowing them to collapse. Clearly these common diseases, all producing airways obstruction, are extremely different in pathogenesis.

Chronic bronchitis

Chronic bronchitis is an extremely common disease, characterized by cough and excessive production of sputum. Estimates of the prevalence of the disease vary but surveys carried out in general practices indicate that approximately 15 per cent of men and 8 per cent of women may suffer from the symptoms. Chronic bronchitis is defined by the World Health Organization as 'a persistent cough with excessive production of sputum for 3 or more months in the year during 3 successive years'. The basic structural change is an alteration in the mucosal lining of the bronchi. This becomes thicker and the proportion of the bronchial wall occupied by the mucosa increases. The ratio of thickness of mucosal layer to total thickness of the bronchial wall is called the Reid index, and in chronic bronchitis it is greater than 30–35 per cent. The increase in the thickness of the mucosal layer is brought about by the increase in number of mucus-secreting cells (goblet cells) and an increase in their size (Fig. 3.1). The goblet cells also spread through the airways and are present in the bronchioles, where they are not found in health. The thickened mucosa narrows the lumen of the airways, which are also blocked by the presence of excessive mucus (which accounts for the persistent productive cough).

Why do these changes come about in the mucosal lining of airways? Most of the evidence about the aetiology of chronic bronchitis comes from large-scale epidemiological studies. The study of large numbers of individuals has been made easier because chronic bronchitis is defined in terms of symptoms. A questionnaire has been developed by the Medical Research Council, posing

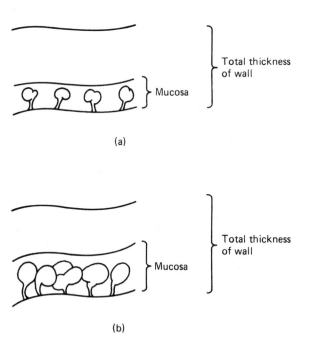

(a)

(b)

Fig. 3.1 Reid index: changes in the bronchial mucosa in chronic bronchitis. (a) Normal. (b) Chronic bronchitis; note the increased size and number of glands in the mucosa of the chronic bronchitic.

standard questions concerning cough, sputum production and shortness of breath. Use of this respiratory questionnaire and a simple test of airways function (peak expiratory flow rate or FEV_1) has made possible large-scale studies of the symptoms of chronic bronchitis and the decline in lung function with time both in normal subjects and in those who have chronic bronchitis.

Aetiology

1. Cigarette smoking. This is by far the most important factor, and tends to dominate any survey in adults. The incidence of the disease in smokers and non-smokers is compared in Fig. 3.2.

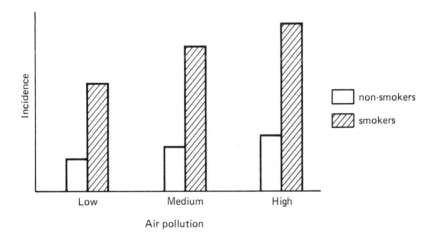

Fig. 3.2 Effect of air pollution and cigarette smoking on the incidence of chronic bronchitis.

2. Air pollution. As shown in Fig. 3.2, this factor operates with cigarette smoking. It has become less important in Britain since the Clean Air Act of 1956.

3. Social class. A preponderance of those with chronic bronchitis are in social classes 3 and 4 (Registrar General's classification).

4. Factors which operate very early in life, such as a respiratory infection during the first year of life. It is interesting that respiratory infections in the first year of a child's life are commoner in the children of smokers.

Chronic bronchitis is very common in Britain, and this disease remains an essentially 'English disorder' (Fig. 3.3). Very careful longitudinal studies of smokers over many years have suggested that a group of smokers can be recognized whose airways are being damaged (about 20 per cent of smokers). The FEV_1 declines with age in everyone, but in some smokers a more rapid rate of fall can be defined (Fig. 3.4); these comprise the susceptible individuals

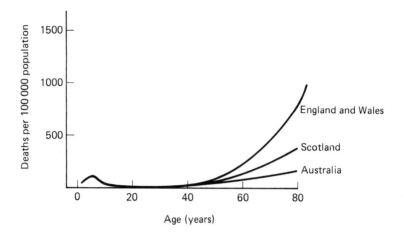

Fig. 3.3 Mortality from bronchitis in England and Wales, Scotland and Australia.

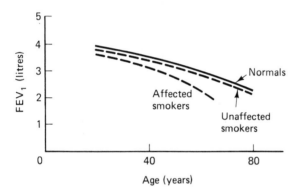

Fig. 3.4 Decline in FEV$_1$ in normal individuals and in smokers, with age (adapted from Fletcher et al., 1976).

who will go on to develop airways obstruction. They, in particular, must stop smoking. It is, of course, only of value to identify the individuals if we can be sure that there are effective methods of deterring them from smoking.

Clinical features

Once the aetiology and structural changes of chronic bronchitis have been described, it is easy to predict the functional outcome of the disease and its effects on the patient. Typically the patient will be a middle-aged heavy smoker (now that smoking is increasing in women, the preponderance of males may become less). By the time of presentation he will complain of a persistent cough producing white (mucoid) sputum and of shortness of breath on exertion. Colds will 'go to his chest', and during periods of respiratory infection he will produce yellow (purulent) sputum. Examination of the patient early in the disease will reveal only wheezes and crackles over the lungs. Cyanosis due to arterial hypoxaemia will only appear late in the progression of the disease. Spirometry will reveal an obstructive pattern which does not respond significantly to a bronchodilator (i.e. the change in FEV_1 will be less than 15 per cent). The progress of the disease is charted by the progress of the airways obstruction, which leads eventually to hypoxaemia and, in some individuals, to hypercapnia. This is the stage of respiratory failure which is discussed in Chapter 5.

Emphysema

Chronic bronchitis and emphysema usually occur together. This is because the most important aetiological factors are shared—that is, cigarette smoking and air pollution. It is very difficult to quantify the degree of emphysema during life, as histological study of the lungs is needed for a final diagnosis. This is because emphysema is defined in terms of a pathological process altering structure. This inevitably makes it difficult to be precise about the diagnosis during life. Emphysema is described as a process leading to an increase in the volume of the air spaces distal to the terminal bronchioles with destruction of alveolar tissue.

When a lung from a patient who has suffered from emphysema is examined, the distribution of the disease anatomically through the lung falls into two divisions:

1. Centrilobular, in which form the centre of the affected lobule is destroyed but many of the other alveoli remain normal. In this way the distribution of ventilation may be grossly distorted even though the total involvement of lung tissue is relatively small.

2. Panlobular (panacinar) emphysema. The distribution in this form is more extensive, most of the alveoli within the lobule being destroyed.

Because of the variation in distribution it becomes difficult to equate functional effects with the amount of tissue involved.

Aetiology

In general, the aetiological factors are the same as those for bronchitis and the two disease processes will be found together. Again, the importance of smoking cannot be overemphasized.

In the case of emphysema there are, however, additional clues as to causation. A group of patients exist with severe panlobular emphysema presenting rather younger than is usual (30–40 years of age). These patients have been found to be lacking in a normal constituent of the plasma proteins, an antiproteolytic substance, α_1-antitrypsin. The connection between this deficiency and emphysema may be elucidated by an animal experiment in which emphysema can be produced by the introduction of papain (which is a proteolytic enzyme) into the trachea. The essential puzzle is to connect cigarette smoking, absence of α_1-antitrypsin in some patients with emphysema and papain-induced emphysema in animals. A possible hypothesis can be constructed. In cigarette smokers macrophages can be observed around the airways. Release of proteolytic enzymes from the macrophages, perhaps as a result of cigarette smoking, may destroy lung tissue. This would be opposed by the presence of α_1-antitrypsin. Possibly cigarette smoking itself may reduce the effectiveness of its antiproteolytic activity, and, of course, its absence would allow proteolytic destruction of the lung to proceed apace.

Altered physiology and clinical presentation

If emphysema is a disease which destroys lung tissue distal to the terminal bronchioles, how does it come to be a disease which produces airways obstruction? The essential reason behind this is that emphysema is a disease destroying the walls of the air spaces and, with it, the support of the airways. In the emphysematous lung the unsupported airways are floppy and will tend to collapse. Because the airways are supported they are held open at high lung volumes and tend to collapse at low lung volumes. This relationship is illustrated in Fig. 3.5, where airways resistance is shown to vary with lung volume, increasing at low lung volumes and decreasing as TLC is approached. If airways function in a patient with emphysema is assessed by means of spirometry this effect will be accentuated, airways collapse being brought about by the forced exhalation. Thus, an obstructive pattern will be produced on spirometry and emphysema becomes classified among the diseases causing airways obstruction. Accordingly, in Table 2.4 emphysema is described as a primary alveolar disease with secondary effects on the airways. Once this is appreciated, it becomes easy to understand why patients with emphysema behave differently from those with chronic bronchitis even though superficially the two diseases produce airways obstruction and share aetiological factors.

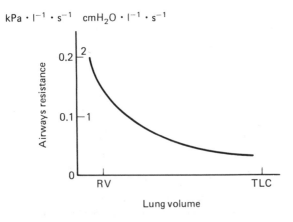

Fig. 3.5 Relationship between airways resistance (R_{aw}) and lung volume. (NB. At high lung volumes airways are held open, so resistance is low.)

Patients with emphysema characteristically present later in life (55–65 years) than those with chronic bronchitis. The presenting symptom is usually severe and disabling shortness of breath. Cough and the production of sputum are not such pronounced features. On examination it is clear that the slightest effort (undressing, for example) causes shortness of breath. Since emphysema is characterized by an increase in the peripheral air spaces, it is not surprising that the chest is found to be overexpanded and hyper-resonant to percussion The lung fields on auscultation are usually quiet, with unremarkable breath sounds.

Usually, chronic bronchitis and emphysema coexist and the clinical presentation will be a mixed one; in spite of this, certain features will suggest the presence of advanced emphysema while certain other features will suggest chronic bronchitis. Clinical examination and the history may give some clues. Tests of lung function will reveal airways obstruction in both groups and there will be an increase in lung volumes in the emphysematous patients, but most markedly a decrease in the transfer factor and transfer coefficient (loss of alveolar surface area in emphysema will have a great effect on this variable). Differences in the appearance of the chest x-ray are beyond the scope of this book but they may be summarized by stating that the chest x-ray in emphysema reflects the consequence of tissue destruction and increased lung volumes. The lungs appear overexpanded, pushing the diaphragm down so that it is flat. The lung fields lack the usual markings and vessels because of the loss of tissue. The attempt to distinguish between bronchitis and emphysema is not important in practical terms for treatment and management, but it does outline how the different pathological processes produce different alterations of function.

Although chronic bronchitis and emphysema usually coexist and the attempt to distinguish patients with chronic bronchitis from those with emphysema will be inexact without full study of the histology of the lungs, it is an established and useful practice to describe two different clinical pathways in patients with severe airways obstruction. These may be equated with the clinical history of patients with emphysema as opposed to those with chronic bronchitis. This is sometimes made a controversial point, because, as has been stressed at some length, one cannot be certain in life how much chronic bronchitis or emphysema a patient has. Perhaps it is best to describe these different modes of presentation and remember that the correlation between structure and function is unfortunately a rather loose one.

'Pink puffers' and 'blue bloaters'

These picturesque terms are used to describe two types of respiratory patient. It is an important distinction because it has implications for treatment and the way in which an individual may respond to an increase in airways resistance.

Pink puffers

Most of these patients can be shown eventually to have severe emphysema. Extreme dyspnoea is the major symptom whilst examination and lung function testing reveal the changes associated with emphysema. The important feature of this syndrome is that estimation of the arterial blood gas tensions reveal a P_{O_2} close to normal and a P_{CO_2} which is typically reduced. Because the arterial hypoxaemia is insufficient to cause cyanosis, the patient appears pink. This is achieved by a high level of total ventilation; hence the patient is pink and puffing.

Blue bloaters

This patient usually presents with a history of chronic bronchitis. The important finding is that he is deeply cyanosed and oedematous—hence blue and bloated. The clue to the development of this situation is found in the arterial blood gases, for the P_{O_2} is reduced (6.7–8 kPa; 50–60 mmHg) and the P_{CO_2} raised (8–8.7 kPa; 60–65 mmHg). As described in Chapter 2, this has been produced by two processes. First, widespread airways disease has led to mismatch of ventilation and perfusion, but in these patients the appropriate response of an increased level of ventilation has not occurred. Mismatch of ventilation and perfusion will lead to a reduced P_{O_2} but, because of an appropriate increase in ventilation, the P_{CO_2} should be held at normal levels or even reduced. The important implication in these patients is that the control mechanism which adjusts the arterial P_{CO_2} is no longer working.

Once arterial hypoxia is established, the rest of the clinical presentation of a blue bloater becomes easy to explain. Arterial hypoxia will lead to an increase in the red cell mass and to pulmonary vasoconstriction. An increase in the pulmonary vascular resistance leads first to hypertrophy of the right ventricle and eventually to permanent changes in the structure of the pulmonary vessels (see Chapter 6). The end-point of this sequence is the development of congestive cardiac failure accompanied by a raised jugular venous pressure, peripheral oedema and evidence of right ventricular hypertrophy. The clinical picture is now that of a blue and bloated patient; recognition of this patient is important because there are important implications for treatment. These are discussed in Chapter 5.

At this point it is of interest to enquire how this condition comes about. In a normal subject this degree of hypoxia accompanied by hypercapnia would produce a distressing increase in ventilation. Why does the blue bloater tolerate such a degree of hypoxia and hypercapnia? Clearly the control of ventilation in these patients can no longer maintain normal oxygenation and removal of CO_2. The analysis of this problem is complex. Perhaps the altered mechanics limit the patient's ability to ventilate even though 'respiratory drive' may be normal. This does not always seem to be the case and investigation reveals subjects who genuinely 'won't breathe' as opposed to those who 'can't breathe'. There remain two possible hypotheses:

1. As lung function declines (mainly an increase in airway resistance), the respiratory control system adapts so that a fall in P_{O_2} and a rise in P_{CO_2} are tolerated.

2. This is a more complicated hypothesis which depends on the observation that the respiratory responses to hypoxia and hypercapnia in normal people vary from individual to individual, some having a considerable change in ventilation for a given increase in P_{CO_2} or fall in P_{O_2} while others scarcely

respond. Potentially those with poor or absent ventilatory responses may be at risk should they develop airway disease. Small alterations in ventilation and perfusion matching during the early disease produce tolerated changes in P_{O_2} and P_{CO_2}. The advance of the disease produces eventually, by the pathway described, a blue and bloated patient.

This remains speculative and emphasizes that we are unable to explain the final physiological consequences of a very common disease process.

Asthma

Asthma brings about an increase in airways resistance by a different mechanism to chronic bronchitis or emphysema, namely bronchoconstriction. (The mechanisms controlling tone in the bronchial smooth muscle have been discussed in Widdicombe and Davies: *Respiratory Physiology*, Chapter 8). Asthma is characterized by an active bronchoconstriction, and the airways of an asthmatic may be regarded as hyper-reactive; they are sometimes referred to as 'twitchy' airways. Any one of a number of stimuli may cause broncho-constriction; see Table 3.1 for a list of so-called trigger factors. Broncho-constriction is undoubtedly the mechanism of a *simple* asthma attack.

Table 3.1 Trigger factors in asthma

Allergic factors	Emotion
pollens	Night time
house dust	
house dust mite	Fumes (e.g. SO_2)
Aspergillus spores	Chemical irritants
animal fur/hair	
Exercise	
Cold air	
Coughing	
Laughter	
Deep breaths	

Sometimes other factors may contribute to the airways narrowing; for example, infected mucus or possibly swelling of the bronchial mucosa. Asthma is defined as variable airways obstruction, the variation occurring with respect to treatment or time. Demonstration of variation in airways resistance is essential to the diagnosis. It is possible that the presence of asthma could be diagnosed by demonstrating that the airways are hyper-reactive. Techniques are now commonly in use to provoke changes in airways resistance by means of bronchial challenge. The subject inhales increasing doses of a bronchoconstrictor substance, methylcholine or histamine, until a 20 per cent fall in FEV_1 is provoked. Asthmatics, with hyper-reactive airways, will produce bronchoconstriction at a much lower dose than normals (Fig. 3.6). It remains to be seen how useful this concept will be. What, for example,

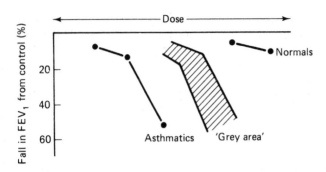

Fig. 3.6   Bronchial hyper-reactivity. Changes in FEV_1 with varying dose of a provoking agent (histamine or methacholine). In asthmatics a 20% fall in FEV_1 is produced by a much smaller dose.

is the relationship between an increased reactivity, variation in airways resistance and the symptoms of asthma? Is increased bronchial reactivity a *constant* hallmark of the asthmatic? The answers to these questions are not yet known but the concept of hyper-reactivity is probably our closest approach to the basic abnormality in asthma.

Although a variety of trigger factors (Table 3.1) are recognized, asthma is usually classified into two types—extrinsic and intrinsic. These categories are of some value in practical terms because they influence treatment.

Extrinsic asthma

This is the best understood form of asthma and constitutes the popular concept of the disease. Characteristically it appears in youth or early adult life and the bronchoconstriction occurs as a result of exposure to one or more inhaled allergens. There is very often a family history of asthma or a related allergic condition (rhinitis or eczema), and the patient may give a clear history indicating the responsible allergens. This group of asthmatics can usually be shown to have positive skin prick tests to the appropriate allergens: perhaps a preferable title for the group would be 'skin-prick-test-positive asthma'. The general rule that asthmatics who develop the disease early in life are skin-prick-test-positive and those developing asthma later in life have negative skin tests is a good approximation. Patients who have positive skin tests are said to be atopic. Approximately 30 per cent of the population are atopic (not all atopic subjects are asthmatic).

The prevalence of asthma of all types is difficult to assess but it may be close to 1 per cent. The presence of atopy in an individual is related to the finding in the plasma of an increased level of the immunoglobulin IgE; it is present in very low concentrations in normal Caucasian subjects, but in atopic subjects the concentration is greatly increased. This is genetically determined and may vary between racial groups. IgE specific to certain allergens can be detected using a specialized technique, the radioallergosorbent test (RAST). This is, of course, firmer proof that a given allergen is involved but the test is expensive and not often necessary clinically (skin tests usually suffice). The mechanism relating allergen exposure, IgE and bronchoconstriction is now relatively well understood. Once the individual has made the IgE, it becomes attached to the surface membrane of mast cells. When the allergens combine with the surface IgE, a change occurs in the mast cell membrane and the cell discharges its granules containing the chemical substances which, in the lung, produce bronchoconstriction. The nature of the change in the mast cell membrane is probably related to changes in Ca^{2+} permeability, allowing an influx of Ca^{2+} which triggers discharge of the granules. The substances released from the mast cells are histamine, bradykinin, a product of arachidonic acid called slow-reacting substance (SRS-A, a mixture of leukotrienes) which produces prolonged smooth muscle contraction and other active substances such as eosinophil chemotactic factor and platelet-activating factor. These produce, in the skin (during skin tests) weal and flare, and, in the lung, bronchoconstriction.

Just as skin tests are used to provoke a reaction in the skin, inhalation challenge can be used to provoke a reaction in the lung. This is sometimes justified if it is necessary to establish that a certain allergen is responsible, and can be important when an individual develops asthma because of exposure to a substance at work and his livelihood may be threatened. The appearance of the skin response may be immediate or delayed; similarly, the broncho-constriction may be immediate, delayed or even a dual response showing both components. This is illustrated in Fig. 3.7, where the changes in airways

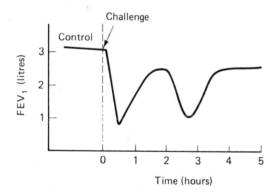

Fig. 3.7 Bronchial challenge: immediate and delayed fall in FEV_1.

function have been monitored by repeated measurements of FEV_1. The immediate response is due to a type I immune response, and the delayed response (occurring some 3–6 hours later) is probably caused by a type III immune response with activation of the complement system.

Since the mechanisms responsible for extrinsic asthma are quite well understood, several approaches for treatment become apparent.

Treatment of extrinsic asthma

Remove the allergens   This is usually more easily said than done. It may be valuable advice if there is a single definable allergy; e.g. cat fur and the problem can be solved if the patient and cat part company. The commonest allergens in Britain are house dust, the house dust mite, grass pollens and the spores of the fungus *Aspergillus fumigatus.* Attempts to avoid these when multiple allergies are present will be extremely difficult. Sometimes simple measures may help, such as vacuum cleaning mattresses regularly and scrupulous attention to keeping dust down.

Desensitization or hyposensitization   The rationale of this therapy is that, once an allergen has been identified in the patient, it can be administered in repeated small doses over a period and the individual thereby 'desensitized'. This depends on provoking the formation of other antibodies of the IgG class to the allergen. The IgG antibodies will combine with the allergen on subsequent exposure to it, and minimize the amount of allergen which can reach the mast-cell-bound IgE in the lungs. The results of this form of treatment are disappointing except where allergy to grass pollen is the main problem. Desensitization to the house dust mite has never been shown conclusively to be of value.

Block the allergic response pharmacologically   This is now possible since the discovery of the chromones (sodium cromoglycate, SCG; Intal). These are substances which stabilize the mast cell membrane and block the key events which occur between combination of allergen with IgE and the discharge of the mast cell granules. There is no oral preparation available of a chromone which is usefully active in this way, and so SCG must be inhaled. SCG is of no value in reversing an established attack of asthma and must be used prophylactically. Approximately 70 per cent of patients with extrinsic asthma will benefit substantially from this treatment.

Intrinsic asthma

This form of asthma typically appears later in life (50 years onwards) than extrinsic. There is no obvious history of atopy (eczema, rhinitis) and there is no family history. The diagnosis is essentially made by establishing that the patient has asthma and that skin prick testing is negative. It is worth remembering that some atopic asthmatics will present late in life. Reflecting the negative skin tests, an intrinsic asthmatic will have normal levels of IgE. As yet we have no clear indication of the cause of intrinsic asthma. Sometimes patients with intrinsic asthma may give a clear history that an attack is precipitated by exposure to dusts or pollens, yet skin tests are negative. Possibly IgE may be present locally only in the lung; consequently, there would not be a raised plasma IgE and no positive skin tests. If this is so, it is surprising that SCG is usually ineffective in this group of patients (only about 10 per cent receiving any benefit). Because we know of no specific mechanism in this form of asthma, the treatment has to be general. Usually, as a group, intrinsic asthmatics have a more severe disease and eventually warrant treatment with steroids either by inhalation or orally.

Before discussing treatment of asthma in general, we must consider the physiological changes of an asthma attack, in order to define the possible scope for pharmacological interference.

Physiology of an asthma attack

The essential feature of an asthma attack is a constriction of the bronchial smooth muscle, leading to narrowing of the airways and an increase in airways resistance. There is a fall in FEV_1 (see Fig. 3.7, showing this during bronchial challenge), an obstructive spirometric pattern develops and the peak expiratory flow rate falls. Changes in FEV_1 and peak expiratory flow rate are a convenient way of monitoring an attack of asthma. If the attack is moderately severe the airways narrowing leads to air-trapping in the lungs and an increase in RV and FRC. On examination, the chest will appear overexpanded. The other findings on physical examination will be loud wheezes over the lungs. The patient may be severely distressed and frightened, and the accessory respiratory muscles in use.

The widespread bronchoconstriction leads to abnormalities in the distribution of ventilation and there is evidence of regions with a low $\dot{V}_A/\dot{Q}$ ratio; that is, areas which are relatively underventilated and overperfused. Consequently there is a fall in arterial P_{O_2} but in most asthma attacks ventilation remains adequate. The patient is able, therefore, to maintain a normal P_{CO_2}. Often there is hyperventilation and the P_{CO_2} is lower than normal. At this point adequate treatment (see below) may end the attack and the variables discussed return towards normal.

Should the attack continue and become more severe, there will be little problem in detecting this if the appropriate measurements are made. Unfortunately, simple clinical observations, without such measurements, may well fail to detect deterioration. Here lies one of the dangers in assessing and treating asthma. If the asthmatic attack continues, the airways resistance may be maintained or even rise and the degree of hypoxia increase. At some point, and it is not certain what defines this physiologically, the patient may be unable to maintain an adequate level of ventilation in the face of such severe airways resistance. In addition to maldistribution of ventilation interfering with gas exchange, alveolar hypoventilation will cause a further fall in arterial P_{O_2} and the P_{CO_2} will start to rise. This is a sinister event in an asthmatic attack and it becomes life-threatening. As the arterial P_{CO_2} rises, the arterial pH falls and a respiratory acidaemia develops. Clinically this is difficult to detect. Appropriate measurements will reveal a further fall in arterial P_{O_2} and a rise in P_{CO_2}. Clinical assessment without measurements is unreliable; this is because the assessment is biased by the degree of wheeze and the obvious respiratory efforts. When the patient can no longer sustain this effort, breathing becomes quieter and the wheeze less pronounced. If the arterial P_{CO_2} rises high enough (over 12 kPa; over 90 mmHg) it will make the patient drowsy. To simple observation the patient has lost his wheeze, breathing has become less distressing and he falls asleep. Attention may be diverted from the patient and treatment relaxed, leading to the patient's death. It cannot be overemphasized that the rational treatment of asthma cannot be divorced from proper monitoring of the FEV_1 or peak expiratory flow rate and, where indicated, the arterial Po_2 and Pco_2.

Respiratory muscle fatigue

At some point in severe asthma, alveolar hypoventilation may exacerbate the situation as discussed above. It is far from clear what determines this physiologically. One possibility is that fatigue of the respiratory muscles, particularly the diaphragm, may determine when this happens. The respiratory muscles will be severely loaded mechanically in overcoming the resistance to air flow of the narrowed airways. Distension of the chest by air-trapping will cause the muscles to work at a mechanical disadvantage; for example, the diaphragm will be flattened. The biochemical events in the muscle which lead to contractile failure are disputed. Changes in the electromyogram (EMG) may indicate the onset of muscle fatigue but this also is the subject of controversy.

Treatment

The majority of mild asthmatic attacks will respond to use of a bronchodilator by inhalation. With the advent of the selective β-stimulant drugs (salbutamol, terbutaline, orciprenaline) which primarily affect airways (β_2 receptors) with minimal effects on cardiac receptors (β_1), effective treatment is readily available. Proper use of an inhaler is difficult and it is worth stressing that teaching the patient how to use an inhaler must be a routine.

In retrospect, it appears that the increased mortality from asthma in the 1960s correlated with the introduction and widespread use of non-specific β-stimulant drugs in pressurized aerosols. These drugs had effects both on the airways and on the heart, and the dangers from their use in asthma were twofold. First, if severe hypoxia is present during the asthma attack, use of a non-selective β-stimulant drug can lead to cardiac arrythmias. Second, it was noted that use of these agents could lead to a further fall in arterial Po_2. As a rule this was about 0.7 kPa (5 mmHg) but larger falls of 1.3–2 kPa (10–15 mmHg) were reported; this could, of course, be extremely important if the patient was already hypoxic. The reason for this is probably due to the β_1 actions of the drug, causing—by an effect either on the heart or on the pulmonary vessels—an increased perfusion of poorly ventilated areas of lung. This would produce a fall in arterial Po_2. Introduction of selective β_2 stimulants has minimized this effect.

If asthma attacks are relatively rare in a patient, treatment with a broncho-dilator alone may suffice. If the attacks are more frequent, regular prophylactic use of the bronchodilator may give adequate control, but in all probability other regular prophylactic treatment will be needed. It is the aim of treatment to keep the patient free from asthma attacks and also to allow him to lead a normal life with airways function maintained as near normal as possible.

In patients with extrinsic asthma regular treatment with SCG, as described, will often give adequate control. In those patients with uncontrolled extrinsic asthma, intrinsic asthma or a life-threatening attack of asthma, treatment will depend on the use of steroids—administered by inhalation, orally or intravenously.

Inhaled steroids

This advance in therapy depends on the use of a steroid preparation (such as beclomethasone dipropionate, Becotide) which is active in the lung when administered by inhalation; it is so active topically that only a very small dose is needed. The absorbed fraction is, therefore, insufficient to cause problems. In this way the benefit of the local effect is obtained without the side effects of systemic steroid therapy. For the chest physician this seems too good to be true; nevertheless clinical experience bears this out. In the doses usually administered by inhalation (up to 800 μg per day, one 'puff' being 50 μg) there are no detectable changes in circulating steroid levels, and consequently no pituitary–adrenal suppression. Inhaled steroids can be used as a substitute for oral doses of 7.5-10 mg of prednisone daily. Like all therapy by inhalation, it will be less effective when there is marked airways obstruction. For this reason it is often effective to precede the inhalation of steroid with a bronchodilator. Inhaled steroids are most often used:

1. For patients with extrinsic asthma who cannot be controlled by SCG and bronchodilators.

2. For intrinsic asthmatics, in whom they are the treatment of choice.

Oral and intravenous use of steroids

Steroids are used systemically in asthma only when the disease is severe. This is usually confined to two situations:

1. Chronic uncontrollable asthma which has not responded to the simpler regimens outlined above and which is interfering unacceptably with the patient's life. In this case the object is to obtain the best 'buy' in terms of symptoms, airways function and dose of steroids. The essential limiting factor comprises the side effects of systemically administered steroids (hypertension, osteoporosis, hypokalaemia, diabetes mellitus, moon face and susceptibility to infection).

2. A severe, life-threatening attack of asthma (often referred to as status asthmaticus). This may be defined as a severe attack of asthma which has not responded to the patient's usual treatment; that is, it has not responded to bronchodilators. It is in this situation that severe arterial hypoxia and even hypercapnia may be found. Treatment is essentially by large doses of steroids. Because the large doses will be used for a short time only, side effects are not a prime concern. In severe life-threatening asthma, doses of 40-60 mg prednisone per day and 200 mg hydrocortisone intravenously every 2 hours are not uncommon. The response of the patient must be monitored by

following the FEV_1 or peak expiratory flow rate and, where necessary, the blood gas tensions. The only side effect of steroids to beware of in this acute situation is hypokalaemia, which must be corrected. When the asthma attack has responded, intravenous steroids may be discontinued and oral steroids withdrawn over 2–4 weeks. The dose of steroids may be adjusted quite simply against the FEV_1 or peak flow rate, whichever variable is monitored.

Undoubtedly steroids can be life-saving in asthma. Unfortunately, the way in which they do this is far from clear. In severe asthma steroids may act in several possible ways:

1. As an 'antiallergic' drug in damping down the allergic reaction responsible.

2. As an 'anti-inflammatory' drug. In severe prolonged asthma the response to steroids may be delayed. If oedema of the bronchial mucosa is involved in narrowing the airways, steroids may reduce this by an anti-inflammatory action.

3. Some action on the β-receptor site. A feature of severe asthma is the loss of responsiveness to β-stimulant bronchodilators. There is evidence that prolonged treatment with steroids in high doses may produce an increase in the number of β-receptor sites. In airways smooth muscle this mechanism may be involved in the regaining of responsiveness to bronchodilators.

Distinguishing between asthma, chronic bronchitis and emphysema

This chapter has been devoted to the clinical features and altered physiology of three diseases which affect airways function. These diseases can usually be distinguished fairly easily on clinical grounds and the results of lung function testing. The major problem which arises is distinguishing some cases of atypical chronic asthma from those of chronic bronchitis and emphysema. This is of some importance because asthma is treatable and the airways disease potentially reversible, which is not so in emphysema or chronic bronchitis as the airways have been structurally damaged. Hence, it is dangerous to label an asthmatic patient as suffering from chronic bronchitis or emphysema, because the same therapeutic efforts will not be made. In some chronic asthmatics the airways obstruction will not be reversed by a bronchodilator and the presence of a chronic productive cough may suggest chronic bronchitis. The distinction between chronic bronchitis and emphysema is largely academic but it is important to pick out patients who may be suffering from chronic asthma. The following points may help in distinguishing these cases:

1. A short history. The patient with chronic bronchitis or emphysema usually has a history of disease for some years; the asthmatic may often give a shorter history of about 2 years.

2. Monitoring peak expiratory flow rate may help (see Fig. 2.9). Although at any one time reversibility may not be present with a bronchodilator, variation in peak flow rate may be apparent. Readings taken in the morning, at mid-day and at night show a considerable diurnal swing (more than 20 per cent variation).

3. Asthma should be suspected when the patient has what appears to be severe emphysema but a normal transfer coefficient. This sometimes indicates severe chronic asthma.

4. The final, and most effective, method of distinguishing asthma may be a trial of steroids in high dosage (prednisone 40–60 mg per day) for up to 2–3 weeks. If this does not produce a significant reversal of the airways obstruction, then in practical terms the patient does not have reversible airways disease. There is much to be said for such a trial of steroids in problem cases, since to miss potentially reversible asthma may be disastrous for the patient.

4

Disease of the lung parenchyma

Chapter 3 described the abnormalities which result from obstruction to the flow of air in the tubes leading to the gas-exchanging surface. These reduce efficiency by limiting air flow and by causing ventilation to be distributed unevenly. This chapter is concerned with the abnormalities resulting from disease of the lung parenchyma itself.

The ways in which the lung tissue can be damaged reflect the stages of the inflammatory reaction. Oedema of the tissue space may be of low protein content, as in the pulmonary oedema of left ventricular disease, or of high protein content as in pneumonia. Infiltration of the tissues by acute inflammatory cells (polymorphonuclear leucocytes and macrophages) takes some hours but it is also readily reversible, whereas involvement in the fibrous reaction of chronic inflammation produces permanent damage.

The consequences of this disruption of the delicate alveolar membrane are:

1. Reduced gas exchange:
   (a) decreased surface area;
   (b) increased length of diffusion pathway;
   (c) uneven distribution of blood in lung.
2. Reduced lung volumes.
3. Stiffening of the lung with distortion:
   (a) reduced compliance;
   (b) increased work of breathing;
   (c) increased transpulmonary pressure changes;
   (d) altered pattern of lung vagal afferent nervous discharge.
4. Interference with the structure of small airways, causing reduced airflow.

The results of these changes are disturbances of blood oxygenation, unproductive cough, heightened sensation of breathlessness at rest and on exercise, and eventually severe disability.

In this chapter the anatomy of the alveoli, its disruption by acute or chronic inflammation of lung parenchyma and the physiological consequences of these changes are discussed.

Anatomy

The structure of the alveolus is described in Widdicombe and Davies (*Respiratory Physiology*, Chapter 1) but a description of the essential features is necessary for the understanding of parenchymal lung disease, so it is repeated here. The majority of the cells of the alveolus are either pulmonary capillary endothelial cells or epithelial cells (very thin inactive type I alveolar cells) supported by a thin basement membrane (Fig. 4.1). The metabolically active type II alveolar cells which normally produce surfactant, and can divide to replace damaged type I cells, are round and not adapted for gas exchange.

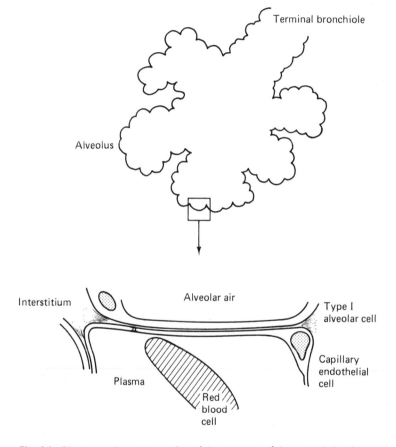

Fig. 4.1 Diagrammatic representation of the structure of the normal alveolus.

The fibrous structure and interstitial tissue of the lung consists of collagen and elastin fibrils, fibroblasts, tissue macrophages and tissue fluid. There is a more substantial fibrous tissue sheath around the bronchial and pulmonary arterial trees. This interconnected fibrous skeleton has two functions: one is to support the alveolar walls, and the other to maintain tension on the walls of the airways holding them open as the lung volume falls. (This is explained below, and see Fig. 4.4.) The interstitital fluid is drained by a system of lymphatics which returns it to the circulation but these channels do not extend into the alveolar tissue. This structure can be disrupted by infiltration with fluid or by solid tissue. Both lead to severe disability of the patient.

Infiltration by fluid

Accumulation of fluid in a tissue can occur in two different ways. It can result from a rise in the pressure of blood in the pulmonary veins leading to a transudate of plasma being forced from vessels, or from release of protein in the tissue which damages the capillary membrane and attracts fluid from the circulation by osmosis forming an exudate.

Transudate

Fluid will accumulate in the tissue spaces of the lung if the tissue drainage mechanisms (transfer of fluid back into the pulmonary capillary or away in the lymphatic system) are overwhelmed by the rate of production. When the pulmonary venous pressure rises, fluid transfer from the lumen of the blood vessels to the tissue space increases. This is protein-poor and is called a transudate of plasma. It accumulates in the interstitial space and then floods into the alveoli. The presence of excess fluid in the lungs leads to changes in the mechanical properties of the lung, to reduced air flow and to altered gas exchange.

Figure 4.2 shows diagrammatically the changes which an increase in lung tissue fluid causes in the alveolar membrane. The tissue space widens, increasing the distance which gas has to diffuse between the alveolar air and the red blood cell; but tissue diffusion distance has to be increased enormously before it becomes the rate-limiting step in gas exchange and this has little effect upon overall gas transfer unless large areas of alveoli are flooded. However, there are other, less obvious, consequences of increased lung tissue fluid which contribute to abnormal lung function. Distortion of the tissue space leads to changes in diameter of the small airways by directly pressing upon them and by reducing the efficiency of the surfactant layer. Excess tissue fluid accumulates around small pulmonary arteries and small airways in a 'perivascular cuff', distorting the walls of the airway and reducing its diameter. It also interferes with the production and distribution of surfactant, allowing surface tension in the airway to rise. When lung volume falls in expiration these airways close, reducing the efficiency of tidal ventilation. The airways may reopen in inspiration as the lung expands, but many remain closed because it may require a transpleural pressure of many centimetres of water to reopen a collapsed airway. If the airway remains closed, the trapped air is absorbed from the alveoli and more extensive segmental collapse follows. Accumulation of fluid in the walls of the small airways contributes to the increase in airways resistance, and the areas of alveolar collapse contribute to the reduction in vital capacity and total lung capacity seen in pulmonary oedema.

More serious for the patient are the changes in the distensibility of the lung which result from interstitial oedema. As the tissue becomes engorged with

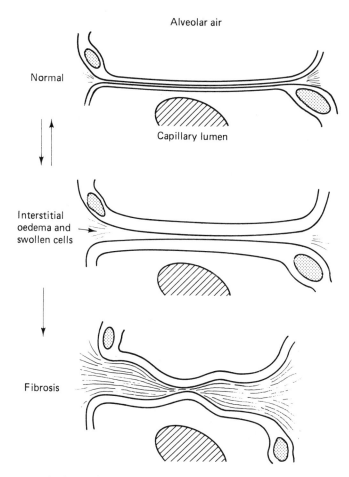

Alveolar air

Normal

Capillary lumen

Interstitial
oedema and
swollen cells

Fibrosis

Fig. 4.2 Anatomical changes associated with interstitial oedema and fibrosis of the lung. The arrows indicate that the changes due to oedema are reversible, whereas fibrosis is permanent.

liquid the fibrous framework is stretched and the compliance of the structure falls. This increases the transpleural pressure changes required to expand the lung and hence the work of breathing. Because vagal afferent discharge is increased by greater intrathoracic pressure swings, stiffer lungs trigger the cough reflex and produce the sensation of breathlessness. These unpleasant effects are magnified by the fact that ventilation/perfusion matching fails and minute ventilation rises. The abnormal gas exchange and rise in minute ventilation are reflected in the arterial blood gas tensions seen in pulmonary oedema when both Pa_{O_2} and Pa_{CO_2} are low (see Chapter 5). The accumulation of fluid in the tissue space disturbs the efficiency and function of the lung, leading to stiff lungs with poor matching of perfusion and ventilation. This is reflected in the disability of patients with pulmonary oedema.

The pulmonary oedema which occurs in patients with disease of the left ventricular muscle illustrates these physiological consequences. Such oedema is most commonly seen following acute myocardial infarction, when the left ventricle pumps inefficiently and pulmonary venous pressure rises. The patient complains of breathlessness, especially on lying flat, and an irritating non-productive cough. The respiratory rate is increased and the patient seems hungry for air. As the minute ventilation rises, wheezy breathing may occur and the peak expiratory flow rate falls. This may cause the unwary doctor to diagnose asthma, and has led to the misleading name 'cardiac asthma'. This cause of wheezing can easily be distinguished from true asthma by examining the patient, when showers of fine crackles are heard over the most dependent parts of the lung as the oedematous airways 'pop' open in inspiration. The chest x-ray shows engorgement of the lymphatic channels and pulmonary veins, areas of alveolar filling and collapse of segments of the lung. The fluid in the lymphatic system in the alveoli is most easily seen in the most dependent part of the lung where the hydrostatic pressure in the pulmonary veins is greatest (Fig. 4.3).

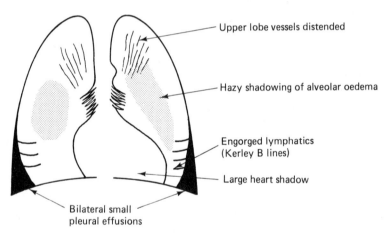

Upper lobe vessels distended

Hazy shadowing of alveolar oedema

Engorged lymphatics
(Kerley B lines)

Large heart shadow

Bilateral small
pleural effusions

Fig. 4.3   Chest x-ray changes in pulmonary oedema caused by disease of the left ventricular muscle.

These changes are induced by fluid distending the tissue of the lung. If the fluid is removed, there is no reason why the structure of the lung should not return to normal and these physiological disturbances disappear. A patient with pulmonary oedema secondary to haemodynamic disturbance illustrates this principle. Correct diagnosis and effective treatment will rapidly restore the lungs to normal, leaving a satisfied physician and an extremely grateful patient.

Exudate

If the excess tissue fluid results from acute inflammation, its characteristics are different. Instead of a transudate of plasma with a low protein content and little cellular infiltrate, it is an exudate rich in protein, acute inflammatory cells and cellular debris. Initially this has the same effects on local lung function as the transudate, but permanent damage to the lung is more likely. In the inflammatory reaction macrophages and polymorphonuclear leucocytes disintegrate, releasing lysozymes rich in enzymes which permeate and attack the lung tissue. If this proceeds without arrest, fibroblastic activity is stimulated and permanent destruction of the architecture of the lung follows. A clinical example of this type of lung reaction is farmer's lung, an acute allergic alveolitis. The subject is allergic to the spores of certain fungi which grow in wet hay (e.g. *Micropolyspora faeni*). When inhaled, the spores settle in the small airways and alveoli, where they are recognized by specific immunoglobulins and the acute inflammatory response is initiated. The random distribution of spores ensures that this is a patchy reaction. If the inhalation of the spores ceases, the reaction subsides. The clinical presentation of this illness is a mixture of acute toxic illness due to the products of inflammation being released into the systemic circulation (fever, malaise and loss of appetite) and the disturbances of lung physiology (breathlessness, dry cough, showers of inspiratory crackles on auscultation of the chest). On removal of the stimulus the subject recovers, the fever subsides, the appetite returns and breathlessness abates. After repeated episodes the respiratory reserve is reduced and the lungs remain permanently small and stiff because pulmonary fibrosis develops. This is the condition often referred to as restriction or restrictive lung disease, and is called diffuse interstitial fibrosis of the lung.

Diffuse interstitial fibrosis

This is the end-product of many episodes of inflammation of the lung, from whatever cause. Diffuse fibrosis of the lung parenchyma distorts normal structure, thickening the alveolar membrane, shrinking and stiffening the lungs and pulling the alveolar spaces into large cystic spaces. This is called honeycomb lung by pathologists or end-stage lung by clinicians, and these names allude to the severity of the physiological disturbance produced by the condition.

Fibrosis of the lung follows acute inflammation centred on the air passages, the alveoli or the pulmonary vessels. The final common pathway to its development is the destruction of the normal architecture of the lung by the acute inflammatory process. If this is induced by an inhaled antigen, it is a patchy condition depending upon the deposition of antigen in the air spaces. If it is associated with circulating antigen, the damage is centred upon the pulmonary vessels and is distributed according to regional pulmonary blood flow. The inflammatory process stimulates fibroblast multiplication and the production of collagen. When this fills the expanded interstitial space, the changes induced by acute inflammation become irreversible and removal of the antigen does not restore the lung to its normal state. As the collagen matures it contracts, shrinking, distorting and stiffening the lung. This is reflected by the measured lung volumes and compliance, all of which fall. Airways are pulled open by the contracting collagen and air flow obstruction is

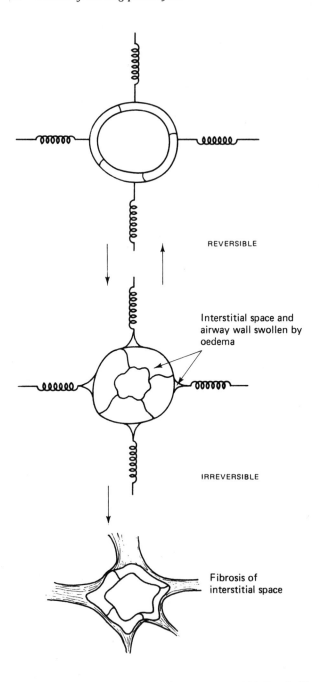

REVERSIBLE

Interstitial space and
airway wall swollen by
oedema

IRREVERSIBLE

Fibrosis of
interstitial space

Fig. 4.4 Airways in pulmonary oedema and interstitial fibrosis. The tissue support loses its elasticity, becomes rigid and distorts the airways. The springs represent the tissue support of the airways.

not seen. Figure 4.4 represents the alterations in airways structure occurring in oedema and fibrosis, and illustrates the way in which interstitial fibrosis pulls the airways open, splinting and distorting them.

The pulmonary capillary bed is also distorted by interstitial fibrosis, causing a fall in the pulmonary capillary volume and mismatch of perfusion with ventilation. Both reduce the efficiency of gas exchange already compromised by the thickening of the alveolar membrane. The lungs are small, stiff and inefficient.

A clinical example of this process is provided by silicosis, a condition caused by the inhalation of dust containing silica, which causes a low-grade inflammatory process and leads to extensive fibrosis. It is often seen in quarriers, sand blasters and coal miners, especially where coal is mined from rock rich in silica (e.g. South Wales). Asbestosis, the pulmonary fibrosis caused by inhalation of asbestos dust, is similar and industrial compensation may be claimed for both conditions. The principal complaint of the patient is breathlessness. Initially this is noticed only on severe exercise, but as the lungs are progressively affected the breathlessness occurs on mild exercise, and eventually on such trivial tasks as getting out of bed or washing. As the lungs become damaged a cough develops. In smokers this occurs early and produces discoloured sputum. The relative roles of smoking and silica inhalation in causing the lung damage are much debated, but it is agreed that smoking hastens its development. As symptoms progress, measured lung function deteriorates. The vital capacity falls, as does the FEV_1, but as both change by about the same proportion the ratio FEV_1/FVC is nearly 100 per cent. The total lung capacity, vital capacity, functional residual capacity all fall. The ability to transfer carbon monoxide from a test breath (transfer factor or transfer coefficient) is low. This disturbance of gas transfer is reflected in the arterial blood gases. The partial pressure of oxygen and of carbon dioxide both fall, indicating hyperventilation and ventilation/perfusion mismatch (see Chapter 5). Hypoxaemia on exercise is severe. The chest x-ray shows diffuse mottling of both lung fields produced by the deposition of collagen in the lung and patches of dense opacity, which are plaques of fibrosis in the lung or on the pleural surface (Fig. 4.5). In asbestosis the degree of pulmonary and pleural fibrosis is extreme. Eventually the lung damage becomes so severe that the victim is housebound and cannot get from room to room without stopping for breath every few paces. These patients may demand and be given supplementary oxygen to breathe but consideration of the lung pathology will indicate why it rarely produces much improvement in exercise tolerance although it may improve the distressing symptom of breathlessness at rest. Severe pulmonary fibrosis is a physiological disaster causing unpleasant disability which progresses relentlessly to death. Wearing masks to prevent inhalation of dust, adequate ventilation of mines or factories and removal of susceptible individuals from exposure are all practised to reduce the risk of those exposed to inhaled dust.

The inhalation of dust is not the only means by which people may develop severe pulmonary fibrosis. In some patients with diseases of the immune system in which the body reacts against its tissues—such as systemic lupus erythematosus or rheumatoid arthritis—the immune system is turned against

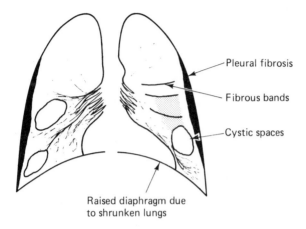

Pleural fibrosis

Fibrous bands

Cystic spaces

Raised diaphragm due
to shrunken lungs

Fig. 4.5   Chest x-ray changes in pulmonary fibrosis.

the tissues of the lung. This leads to the production of circulating antibodies and immune complexes which lodge in the pulmonary capillaries, damaging them and leading to pulmonary fibrosis. Suppression of the inflammatory reaction with corticosteroid drugs (prednisolone) or immunosuppressive agents (cyclophosphamide or azathioprine) is all that can be offered, and sometimes fails to halt the progression of these cases of 'idiopathic' fibrosing alveolitis. In 1944 Hamman and Rich described four patients with pulmonary fibrosis which caused death within a few weeks, and the subsequent 35 years have yielded no treatment which helps patients with this aggressive self-destructive abnormality. Perhaps a better understanding of immune processes and autoimmune disease, with which this condition is strongly linked, will alter our ability to arrest the progress of pulmonary fibrosis or to reverse it, but we await the means to do so.

   The physiological problems of stiff lungs are severe and while the cause of the stiffness is only oedema the condition is reversible. It is important to recognize the problem at this stage, since failure to do so allows fibrosis of the lung to ensue. Prevention of this progression is not always possible, but this should not lull the physician into inactivity since failing to act may result in a permanently breathless disabled patient.

5

Respiratory failure

In Chapter 2 it was pointed out that respiratory failure could be divided, on the basis of the arterial gas tensions, into two types:

1. Hypoxaemia (Pa_{O_2} < 8 kPa; 60 mmHg) accompanied by hypercapnia (Pa_{CO_2} > 6.5 kPa; 49 mmHg).
2. Hypoxia, accompanied by a Pa_{CO_2} either normal or below normal.

The mechanisms which lead to these two distinct forms of respiratory failure are described in Chapter 2. The importance of this classification is that it has implications not only for the likely cause of respiratory failure but also for treatment. This chapter will be largely concerned with the principles of treating respiratory failure. Rational treatment can be planned only if there is a diagnosis. It will be assumed that the first step in diagnosis has established that the patient has respiratory failure and the blood gases are known. This is a reversal of the steps which will usually occur. Usually it will have been established that the patient has a given disease and the second step will reveal, on blood gas analysis, that this is sufficiently severe to have given rise to respiratory failure. Nevertheless, in this chapter we can approach the subject more easily by starting from the findings on blood gas analysis and ask the following questions:

1. If the arterial P_{O_2} is low and the P_{CO_2} high, why is the patient not ventilating adequately?

or

2. If the patient is severely hypoxic but with a normal arterial P_{CO_2}, why is there a defect of pulmonary gas exchange?

Hypoxic, normocapnic respiratory failure

This type of respiratory failure occurs because gas exchange is abnormal. The low, or normal, Pa_{CO_2} reveals that the level of ventilation is adequate or even excessive. The mechanism which most frequently underlies this form of respiratory failure is the mismatching of ventilation to perfusion. A classification and some causes are shown in Table 5.1.

This form of respiratory failure is relatively easy to treat. Appropriate therapy must be aimed at managing the underlying disease process. (To deal

Table 5.1 Mechanisms and causes of hypoxic, normocapnic respiratory failure

Reduced inspired Po_2
  Altitude
  Can happen with faulty breathing apparatus

True shunting (right-to-left shunt)
  Pulmonary AV malformation
  Cyanotic congenital heart disease (i.e. R–L shunt through a ventricular septal defect because of high pulmonary vascular resistance)

Ventilation/perfusion mismatch
  Pulmonary oedema
  Pneumonia
  Chronic bronchitis (if not in stage of CO_2 retention)
  Emphysema
  Asthma
  Pulmonary embolism
  Sarcoid
  Fibrosing alveolitis
  Pneumoconiosis
  Bronchiectasis

with this aspect for all the diseases in Table 5.1 is beyond the scope of this book.) The general treatment will be to increase the inspired O_2 to combat the hypoxaemia. In the presence of a reasonable cardiac output and normal haemoglobin it should suffice to raise the Pao_2 to 8–9.3 kPa (60–70 mmHg). Oxygen therapy is simple in this group of patients because they will tolerate high concentrations of inspired O_2. There is an important caveat. In this context, 'high inspired O_2' means levels up to 40%; above this value, O_2 therapy will, if prolonged, lead to lung damage.

Many masks are available which will provide an inspired O_2 of 40% without significant rebreathing (MC mask, Polymask). If the patient will not tolerate a mask, nasal prongs may prove more successful.

Hypoxic, hypercapnic respiratory failure

The causes of this form of respiratory failure are listed in Table 5.2. The clinical features will vary considerably according to the cause and it is likely that the basic diagnosis will to a large extent determine the treatment. In Chapter 3 the physiological features of this form of respiratory failure were described when the cause was chronic airways obstruction. This is by far the commonest cause of respiratory failure with a raised $Paco_2$, and for this reason discussion of treatment will concentrate mainly on this condition.

Treatment of this form of respiratory failure is more complicated than in the normocapnic form. This is because the raised $Paco_2$ implies that the patient has lost the ability to control this variable. This may occur because the raised Pco_2 is tolerated and, for reasons which we do not understand (see Chapter 3), it does not produce the hyperpnoea which would ensue in a normal subject at this level of hypoxia and hypercapnia. This group of patients comprise those who 'won't breathe' and these are the chronic bronchitics. They are not

Table 5.2 Causes of alveolar hypoventilation (hypoxic, hypercapnic respiratory failure)

Anatomical site	Cause
Brain stem (central 'drive')	Drug overdose: Morphine Barbiturates
Spinal cord	Transection above C3 Poliomyelitis
Peripheral nerves	Peripheral neuropathy (Guillain-Barré syndrome)
Neuromuscular junction	Paralysing drugs (e.g. curare) Myasthenia gravis
Muscles	Myopathy Fatigue of respiratory muscles
Rib cage and chest wall	Multiple fractured ribs Severe kyphoscoliosis
Lungs	Airways obstruction: Asthma Chronic bronchitis

absolutely limited as regards ventilation, and given an adequate stimulus they can usually reduce their $Paco_2$ for a short time. The other group of patients with this form of respiratory failure are those who 'can't breathe'; here there is an absolute inability to ventilate adequately and excrete a CO_2 load. For example, a patient treated with a neuromuscular paralysing agent cannot ventilate and will rapidly develop hypoxia and hypercapnia. This important division determines treatment. In those who 'can't breathe' the rational treatment must be, in most cases, mechanical ventilation. The situation is more complicated in the chronic bronchitics who 'won't breathe'; it is complicated for the following reasons which determine the content of most of this chapter. Although mechanical ventilation will solve the problem in that it enables us to reduce the $Paco_2$ and oxygenate the patient, this is not always appropriate therapy in a chronic bronchitic. This is the end-result of a chronic disease, and mechanical ventilation via an endotracheal tube or tracheostomy is a formidable undertaking for both the patient and the medical staff. Mechanical ventilation is not, therefore, always an appropriate treatment. The problem remains that the patient may have a dangerous level of hypoxaemia and the obvious way to combat this is by increasing the inhaled Po_2.

The problem with oxygen therapy

The chronic bronchitic develops hypoxic, hypercapnic respiratory failure because there are two fundamental defects (see Chapter 3, section on blue bloaters). An imbalance between ventilation and perfusion leads to hypoxaemia, but, since these patients have lost the ability to control the level of Pco_2, this also rises. Because there is $\dot{V}A/\dot{Q}$ imbalance *and* alveolar hypoventilation, not only is the $Paco_2$ raised but also the Pao_2 is lower than it would be if there were only $\dot{V}_A/\dot{Q}$ imbalance. This complicated alteration of normal physiology leaves the patient in a dangerous situation.

If the patient is left breathing room air, death from respiratory failure will supervene because of hypoxaemia. A Pa_{O_2} of 3.3 kPa (25 mmHg) or less, if maintained for any length of time, is usually lethal. At this level of Pa_{O_2}, the Pa_{CO_2} will have risen to almost 12 kPa (90 mmHg). Acutely, this will produce a respiratory acidaemia and a fall in arterial pH. As the Pa_{CO_2} rises, hypercapnia begins to have effects in its own right. These are not sufficiently specific to be of use in diagnosis but they have important consequences. At these levels of Pa_{CO_2} (12 kPa; 90 mmHg) the patient may develop drowsiness proceeding to coma, a flap of the outstretched hands, a coarse tremor, warm peripheries due to dilated cutaneous vessels, cardiac arrythmias and increased intracranial pressure. The most important of these is drowsiness which leads to coma as the Pa_{CO_2} rises over 13.3 kPa (100 mmHg); this is CO_2 narcosis. The manifestations of hypercapnia do not seem to bear a constant relationship to levels of Pa_{CO_2}. They may well be better related to rate of rise of Pa_{CO_2}.

If the patient breathing room air is at risk of dying from hypoxia, the obvious line of treatment is to increase the inhaled O_2 concentration. Once O_2 therapy has been started a new problem arises, for CO_2 narcosis now becomes a real danger. Breathing room air, the patient may die from hypoxia; if the inspired O_2 is supplemented, the patient becomes comatose and may die from CO_2 narcosis. The reason for this will be clarified if Fig. 5.1 is consulted. This should make clear that when breathing room air fatal levels of hypoxia occur with a Pa_{CO_2} of about 12-13.3 kPa (90-100 mmHg). Once O_2 therapy is started, the situation changes drastically. The patient will now encounter

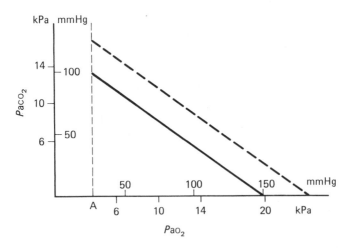

Fig. 5.1 O_2/CO_2 diagram showing the effects of O_2 therapy. The solid line indicates possible combinations of Po_2 and Pco_2 for a patient breathing room air (assuming RQ = 0.8). At point A (Pco_2 circa 13.7 kPa, 100 mmHg) death will occur from hypoxia. The broken line indicates the new relationship if O_2 therapy is started. Narcotic levels of Pco_2 are reached before death from hypoxia (adapted from Campbell, 1965)..

narcotic levels of $P\mathrm{aco_2}$—13.3 kPa (100 mmHg) and over—before death from hypoxia. CO_2 narcosis carries its own dangers, not least because a comatose patient will no longer cough and clear his airways.

There is a further mechanism to be considered. If a patient with chronic bronchitis has developed hypoxia and hypercapnia, the respiratory control system is no longer working as it should. This complicates O_2 therapy further, since increasing the inspired O_2 concentration and hence the $P\mathrm{aco_2}$ can, in some individuals, remove all the drive to breathing. A rapidly rising $P\mathrm{aco_2}$ ensues. The deduction from this must be that patient's ventilation depended entirely on a hypoxic drive; once this is removed, ventilation falls even further and dangerous hypercapnia may develop. Which individual will respond in this way cannot be predicted, nor do we know why the critical drive to breathing in these subjects depends on hypoxia. It may be that it is a residual drive arising from the peripheral chemoreceptors; or, it has been suggested, a critical fall in O_2 availability around the brain stem chemoreceptors may lead to a tissue acidosis. The drive to breathing might thus arise from this central fall in pH which would be remedied by a rise in $P\mathrm{o_2}$. At present this remains a hypothesis.

We are faced with a difficult clinical problem. Left alone, the patient may die of hypoxia; treated appropriately with an increased inspired $P\mathrm{o_2}$, dangerous hypercapnia may ensue. It is fortunate that a true appreciation of physiological principles enables us to deal with this dilemma. The aim of O_2 therapy is not, of course, to return the $P\mathrm{ao_2}$ to normal but to prevent the patient dying from tissue O_2 lack. We must provide enough extra O_2 to keep him away from potentially lethal levels without giving so much as to lead to dangerous respiratory depression. The shape of the O_2 dissociation curve is the key to the solution. At low levels of $P\mathrm{ao_2}$ a small increase will produce a

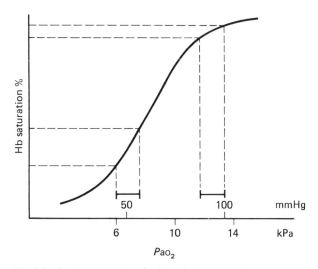

Fig. 5.2 O_2 therapy and the O_2 dissociation curve. For a given rise in $P\mathrm{ao_2}$ (represented by the horizontal bars) there will be a greater increase in Hb saturation at a low $P\mathrm{o_2}$ than at a high $P\mathrm{o_2}$.

large change in haemoglobin saturation (Fig. 5.2). It is possible to negotiate this difficult problem by a compromise; enough O_2 must be given to raise the Po_2 and haemoglobin saturation away from critical levels, while at the same time ensuring that the hypoxic drive to breathing is not completely removed. The decision to initiate O_2 therapy in a patient with hypoxic, hypercapnic respiratory failure will always carry the risk of promoting dangerous hypercapnia. The decision to treat is made on the basis of the Pao_2 and the treatment is monitored by following the $Paco_2$.

The level of Pao_2 at which O_2 therapy should be started is debatable. Patients with chronic bronchitis in this condition usually have a well maintained cardiac output and a raised haemoglobin concentration and red cell mass. The decision can well be made on the level of Pao_2. Certainly at a Pao_2 of 6 kPa (45 mmHg) O_2 therapy becomes desirable, and around 4.7 kPa (35 mmHg) a necessity. The aim is to increase the Pao_2 to levels around 6.7-7.3 kPa (50-55 mmHg) without an uncontrolled rise in $Paco_2$. At this stage it is appropriate to consider how this may be achieved.

Controlled oxygen therapy

Controlled O_2 therapy depends on providing a precise inspired O_2 concentration. The masks described previously in this chapter provide an inspired O_2 of about 40%. Masks have been developed which will provide an inspired O_2 of 24% or 28%. The principle of such a mask (Ventimask) is shown in Fig. 5.3. Oxygen from a cylinder, at a given flow rate, emerges from the nozzle; because of the Venturi effect, air is entrained through the side holes in such a proportion that the final O_2 concentration is fixed. The masks are relatively comfortable to wear and, because of the high flow rate, rebreathing is not a problem. Selection of the appropriate 24% or 28% O_2 mask allows a trial of O_2 therapy at a precise level of raised inspired O_2 concentration. Oxygen therapy must, like any other treatment, be precisely prescribed and the details of type of mask and flow rate entered in the patient's record. It is astonishing how often patients are receiving O_2 without any instruction begin given.

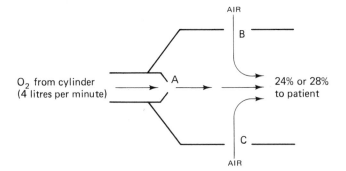

Fig. 5.3 Mask for controlled O_2 therapy. A, the aperture for the O_2 stream; B and C, side holes for entraining air.

Management of controlled oxygen therapy

The effect of O_2 therapy is assessed by measuring the $Paco_2$ some 1-2 hours after the treatment has started. The rise in $Paco_2$ will vary from patient to patient and it is difficult to make predictions. Inevitably, if there is a rise in Pao_2, there will be a rise in $Paco_2$. The danger is a $Paco_2$ which does not stabilize but continues to rise. After 1-2 hours' treatment with 24% O_2 the $Paco_2$ will rise about 0.7 kPa (5 mmHg) and with 28% O_2 about 1.3-2 kPa (10-15 mmHg). With these figures, approximate predictions can be made. In moderately severe respiratory failure ($Paco_2$ 6.7-7.3 kPa, 50-55 mmHg) a rise of 1.3-2 kPa (10-20 mmHg) $Paco_2$ will not be dangerous, whereas in more severe cases ($Paco_2$ 8.7-9.3 kPa, 65-70 mmHg) such a rise will produce dangerous levels of $Paco_2$. Any extra rise will lead to CO_2 narcosis. Clearly in the more severe cases a 24% mask will be used initially. This is probably always safest, a 28% mask being substituted when it has been proved the patient can tolerate 24% O_2.

Other measures used in treating hypoxic, hypercapnic respiratory failure

Controlled O_2 therapy has been described on the assumption that the patient will be suffering from an exacerbation of chronic bronchitis. Usually the exacerbation will have been precipitated by infection and the patient will be producing thick, purulent sputum. For most of the conditions listed in Table 5.2, mechanical ventilation (see below) will be more important once hypercapnia has developed.

In chronic bronchitis with hypercapnic respiratory failure other steps are essential in addition to O_2 therapy. They are, in probable order of importance:

1. *Physiotherapy.* This is probably as important as O_2 therapy. Regular physiotherapy will clear infected sputum from the airways and improve gas exchange. Moreover, regular physiotherapy will waken the patient, promote coughing and contribute more than any other single treatment, perhaps, to a successful outcome.

2. *Antibiotics.* If infection has been the precipitating factor in the exacerbation, the likely organisms are *Streptococcus pneumoniae* or *Haemophilus influenzae*. A broad-spectrum antibiotic such as amoxycillin, ampicillin or co-trimoxazole is indicated.

3. *Adequate hydration.* If the patient is severely ill and drowsy, it is unlikely that he will have had an adequate fluid intake. Rehydration is important, but, in view of the possible presence of congestive cardiac failure, care must be taken to avoid fluid overload.

Finally, severe hypoxia over many years, now complicated by an acute exacerbation, may have so increased the pulmonary vascular resistance as to lead to right heart failure. The essential measures are to treat the respiratory failure as above. Any therapy aimed at improving the heart failure *per se* must be seen as of secondary importance only. Controlled O_2 therapy combined with these measures will often prove successful, the patient improving over

48–72 hours. If the situation continues to worsen, one further measure is worth discussing before moving on to mechanical ventilation.

Respiratory stimulant drugs

Hypoxic, hypercapnic respiratory failure comes about because of lack of respiratory drive. Respiratory stimulant drugs exist, and on theoretical grounds they should be useful in treating this form of respiratory failure. In practice they are, at most, of marginal value only. This may be because the drugs available are not specific respiratory stimulants, but analeptics with widespread actions on the central nervous system. It is also asking a lot of a drug to reverse an abnormality of respiratory control when we have no precise knowledge of the origin of this abnormality. The dose of most respiratory stimulant drugs which will have an effect on breathing is close to the toxic dose and may produce agitation, twitching and tremor. Nikethamide is such an analeptic with these properties; one of the earliest drugs used as a respiratory stimulant, it is still occasionally of value.

Perhaps the respiratory stimulant drugs should not be viewed as agents for lowering the $Paco_2$ but rather as an adjunct to controlled O_2 therapy. If controlled O_2 therapy with 24% O_2 promotes an unacceptable rise in $Paco_2$, it may be possible to use a respiratory stimulant drug—not to lower the $Paco_2$ but to enable the continuation of O_2 therapy and prevent a further rise. Alternatively, use of such a drug may allow 28% O_2 to be given rather than 24% O_2 without further rise in $Paco_2$.

Probably the most effective and commonly used respiratory stimulant (after regular physiotherapy!) is doxapram. Doxapram has a direct effect on the peripheral chemoreceptors and a direct central action on the brain stem centres. It is administered intravenously as a constant infusion in doses ranging from 0.5 to 4.0 mg per minute. The dose infused may be varied while the effect on arterial blood gases is monitored. The side effects of the drug are tremor, agitation, and a burning sensation in the perineum.

If the use of a respiratory stimulant drug can halt a rise in $Paco_2$ during O_2 therapy, this is an important contribution. The only alternative may be mechanical ventilation, and this is a form of treatment which should not be lightly undertaken.

Mechanical ventilation

The decision to take over a patient's ventilation mechanically is a major one; it is a skilled technique and should be undertaken only where there is adequate experience available. It is extremely difficult to be dogmatic about the indications for mechanical ventilation. Table 5.2 shows that there are a large number of reasons for alveolar hypoventilation, and the decision to start mechanical ventilation will obviously vary with the underlying cause. Mechanical ventilation is not limited to these conditions; it may sometimes be employed for patients with severe hypoxic, normocapnic respiratory failure. It will be used in these patients when the hypoxaemia is dangerous and the distress of hyperventilation is overwhelming the patient. For example, mechanical ventilation is sometimes employed in severe pulmonary oedema (even though the $Paco_2$ may be low because of excessive ventilation).

Perhaps the easiest way to classify the indications for mechanical ventilation is to consider the clinical contexts in which it is likely to become necessary.

Acute illness Mechanical ventilation is necessary because without it the patient will die. This may be obvious because the patient has stopped breathing, because the arterial gases have reached life-threatening levels or because the effort involved in breathing is too much to be sustained (see section on respiratory muscle fatigue, Chapter 3). These limits may be reached in such conditions as severe head injury, drug overdose, trauma to the chest or lungs and pulmonary oedema (including adult respiratory distress syndrome, 'shock lung'). The indication for starting mechanical ventilation is the patient's immediate survival. Sometimes the basic diagnosis may not be known, but once mechanical ventilation has been started further steps can be taken to determine the underlying problem (e.g. head injury or drug overdose). This approach will often occur in the emergency room.

Chronic illness Whereas the decision to start mechanical ventilation (described above) is mandatory, in chronic disease it will be an elective decision. We can subdivide this into two ways in which the elective decision can arise:

1. An elective decision made before the onset of respiratory failure (as judged from the blood gases). This will often happen in the course of a chronic neuromuscular disorder such as a peripheral neuropathy involving the nerves to the respiratory muscles or a disease involving the respiratory muscles themselves. Here, the concern is to start mechanical ventilation before respiratory failure occurs; that is, before the patient develops hypoxia or hypercapnia. Often the decision will be determined by the patient's inability to protect his airway. This may happen because the disease removes the ability to cough (e.g. a bulbar palsy) or because the fall in respiratory function makes coughing an inefficient process (i.e. there may not be enough muscle power or enough gas volume). If food and secretions cannot be cleared from the airways, then the airways must be protected either by passing a cuffed endotracheal tube or by forming a tracheostomy. Once this has been done, the decision to attach a mechanical ventilator can be undertaken electively, and before the onset of significant hypoxia or hypercapnia.

2. An elective decision after the onset of respiratory failure. This will occur in the course of severe airways obstruction and the patient will be suffering from asthma or chronic bronchitis:

(a) In asthmatics this decision is forced when the patient can no longer ventilate adequately against such an increase in airways resistance. This will become clear because of the patient's increasing discomfort, signs of circulatory decompensation, a falling Pa_{O_2} and a rising Pa_{CO_2}. In asthmatics the decision to undertake mechanical ventilation is easier because the situation is potentially reversible. Occasionally an asthmatic will fall into the category 'acute illness' described above and present *in extremis*, requiring immediate mechanical ventilation. Mechanical ventilation of an asthmatic is technically extremely difficult because of the high inflation pressure required to force air into the lungs. If the minute ventilation is set too high, the inflation pressure needed will interfere with cardiac filling and the patient may die because of a low cardiac output. The compromise is to use as low an inflation pressure and minute volume as possible, remembering that the aim is to maintain oxygenation and remove the fatiguing respiratory effort. It is not essential to return the $Pa\text{CO}_2$ to normal immediately.

(b) In chronic obstructive airways disease the decision is difficult and always requires careful consideration. The aim must be to ventilate only those patients in whom the factors which have precipitated respiratory failure are reversible. Such reversible factors may be oversedation or poorly managed O_2 therapy or sometimes an overwhelming respiratory infection. Here, mechanical ventilation is used to buy time. Mechanical ventilation is to be avoided in those patients who have slowly reached this degree of respiratory failure because of the inexorable progress of their chronic bronchitis. There is no reversible factor and it will be impossible to wean the patient from the mechanical ventilator. Before committing such a patient to mechanical ventilation, with its potential complications, his previous condition and lung function must be taken into account.

Mechanical ventilators are of many different varieties but they work on one of two basic principles:

1. Intermittent positive pressure ventilation (IPPV) via an endotracheal tube or tracheostomy tube. IPPV depends on a positive pressure to inflate the lungs; the degree of positive pressure used and the time over which the pressure is delivered can be varied, as can be the time for expiration. If necessary, a negative expiratory pressure can be applied; this will 'suck' air out. Alternatively, positive end-expiratory pressure (PEEP) may be used in an attempt to prevent airways closure. Using a mechanical ventilator, high concentrations of inspired O_2 can be achieved but it must be remembered that continued use of an inhaled O_2 greater than 40% may damage the lungs.

2. Positive–negative ventilators. These ventilators depend on the application of a negative pressure to the outside of the thorax during the inspiratory phase. This is the ventilator described as an 'iron-lung' (Drinker respirator). The method has the advantages that the upper airways do not have to be interfered with by intubation or tracheostomy. This may be critical in the long-term management of some patients. On the other hand, there is no safety for the airways in the absence of a cuffed tube. The patient must be able to protect his own airways by coughing; vomit, or secretions may be sucked into the lungs in a patient with no cough.

Long-term oxygen therapy
Oxygen therapy has been discussed so far in this chapter in the context of an acute alteration in blood gas tensions. Some patients, who have followed the progress outlined for the blue bloater, may remain chronically in respiratory failure and in a reasonably steady state. The question has been asked whether provision of long-term O_2 therapy will prevent progression of the disease (or even reverse the changes in the pulmonary vasculature) and whether such

treatment will improve the quality of life and reduce morbidity.

Certainly in the short term (O_2 therapy for 1 month) improvements can be measured. Patients with severe chronic bronchitis and hypoxaemia can be shown, after 1 month of O_2 therapy, to have improved in that the packed cell volume and red cell mass are reduced and the pulmonary vascular resistance has fallen. Recently trials have been organized by the Medical Research Council in the UK and by the National Institutes of Health in the USA. These trials have compared, over a number of years in selected patients, regimens of continuous O_2 therapy throughout the 24 hours, O_2 therapy for 15 hours per day and no O_2 therapy. The results show that mortality and morbidity are both improved by O_2 therapy, continuous O_2 being more effective than 15 hours of therapy and 15 hours of therapy having a significant benefit over no O_2 therapy. There is, of course, an additional benefit in 15 hours therapy per day, because for 9 hours of the day the patient can be independent of an O_2 supply. The provision of this treatment is demanding and expensive. The introduction of O_2 concentrators, which use a system of molecular sieves to concentrate O_2 from room air, may allow this treatment to be provided in the home more easily and at less cost.

6

The pulmonary circulation

Chapters 3 and 4 of this book concentrated on the airways and the lung parenchyma. However, the lung would not function as a gas exchanger without an efficient supply of blood. This chapter describes the normal pulmonary circulation, its anatomy and its controlling mechanisms and then considers how disease of the lung disturbs its function. Clinical examples are described, illustrating the effects of these diseases in patients.

The normal pulmonary circulation

Anatomy

The pulmonary circulation consists of a branching system of arteries, the pulmonary capillary bed and the pulmonary veins. The right ventricle ejects systemic venous blood into the main pulmonary artery. This divides into the main pulmonary arteries which supply the right and left lungs. These then divide, forming a branching system which follows the bronchial tree until the pulmonary arterioles deliver the blood into the pulmonary capillary bed. The exchange of oxygen and carbon dioxide occurs between the alveolar air and the pulmonary capillary blood. The oxygenated blood is collected by the pulmonary veins and delivered to the left atrium for distribution through the systemic circulation.

The pulmonary circulation is confined within the thoracic cage and the blood requires a low driving pressure to traverse the capillary bed (see below). This is reflected by the structure of the main pulmonary arteries, which have muscle coats and an elastic lamina but are thin-walled when compared with the vessels of the systemic circulation. As they branch, the vessels maintain their muscular wall and hence their ability to constrict right down the branching system as far as the pulmonary arterioles. The ability of these small vessels to control their diameter has important implications for the distribution of the pulmonary blood flow since the flow of blood of a given viscosity through a vessel is inversely proportional to the fourth power of the radius of the vessel (derived from Poiseuille's law). A small change in the diameter of a small blood vessel has a large effect on blood flow whereas a similar change in a vessel of large diameter will have little effect on flow. The role of the large pulmonary vessels which are distensible and elastic is to receive the pulsatile output of the right ventricle and smooth its flow to the lungs. The role of the small pulmonary vessels is to regulate the blood flow at local level. The pulmonary veins also have muscular walls but it is doubtful if they play any role in the regulation of pulmonary blood flow, acting instead as a reservoir for left atrial filling.

The pulmonary capillary bed is an open matrix of vessels surrounding the alveoli. It is well suited to gas exchange, having a large surface area and thin walls, but the walls have no muscular elements and there appears no possibility of the size of the vessels being actively regulated. The patency of pulmonary capillaries is dependent upon external factors. If the pressure of the alveolar air is higher than the pressure within the pulmonary capillary, the capillary will collapse and flow through it cease. If the capillary is stretched and distorted by the fibrous elements of the interstitial tissue of the lung then blood flow will be reduced. Experiments on an isolated perfused lobe of the lung of a dog show that the pulmonary vascular resistance is higher at very low or very high lung volumes (Fig. 6.1). This observation is explained by the

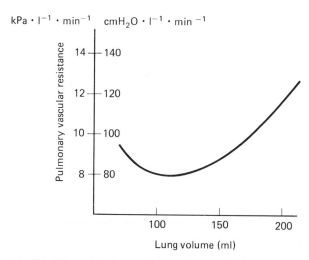

Fig. 6.1 The relation between lung volume and pulmonary vascular resistance in the isolated lung of a dog. (Redrawn, with permission, from J. B. West, 1979, *Respiratory Physiology: the essentials.* Williams & Wilkins, Baltimore.)

hypothesis that lung capillaries are kinked at very low lung volumes and are stretched at high lung volumes. Both would reduce the pulmonary capillary diameter and increase vascular resistance. The relation of pulmonary blood flow to alveolar pressure is discussed below.

Pulmonary artery pressure

Blood flows through the blood vessels from arteries to veins down a pressure gradient. Generating and maintaining a head of pressure is an energy-wasteful process, and the ideal system keeps the pressure to the minimum required to distribute blood to all parts of the circulation and to maintain adequate flow. Because the heart is in the thoracic cage, it is not at the top of the column of blood in the upright human, so pressure in the arterial tree must be sufficient to raise the blood to the highest point. In the systemic circulation the top of the head is about 50 cm above the heart and 180 cm above the feet. If flow is to be maintained in the capillaries of the brain and the feet, the mean arterial pressure must be sufficient to perfuse the top of the column of blood and the resistance to flow in the arterioles of the dependent parts must be high. A low resistance here would allow all the blood to flow through the capillary bed of the legs, dropping the arterial pressure and leading to failure of blood flow in the head. This is what happens to the guardsmen who faint on a hot day. Because the top of the lung is a mere 15 cm above the heart and the pulmonary circulation is only 30 cm from top to bottom, a low driving pressure is possible. The normal pressures of the pulmonary and systemic circulations are shown in Fig. 6.2.

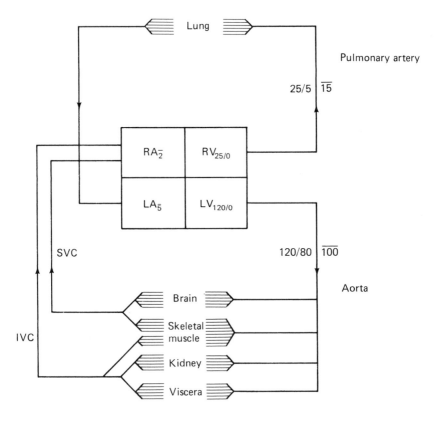

Fig. 6.2 Diagrammatic representation of the circulation, showing the dynamic pressures and mean pressures in the pulmonary and systemic circulation. (All pressures are in mmHg.)

The fact that the entire cardiac output passes through the pulmonary circulation means that any increase in cardiac output must be accompanied by increased pulmonary blood flow. This could be achieved by raising the driving pressure, but reducing the resistance to flow or increasing the size of the capillary bed would allow increased flow for the same driving pressure. In the resting normal human, blood flow in the lungs is unevenly distributed. These differences are greatest in the upright posture, when the apex of the lung receives very little of the pulmonary blood flow (Fig. 6.3) (see Widdicombe and Davies: *Respiratory Physiology*, Chapter 6). Increases in cardiac output can be accommodated for minimal change in driving pressure by recruitment of the areas of underperfused lung. The efficiency of this mechanism is demonstrated by measuring the pulmonary artery pressure in an exercising athlete who raises his cardiac output from 5 to about 20 litres of blood per minute. Under these circumstances the pulmonary artery pressure rises from 25/5 to about 30/10 mmHg.

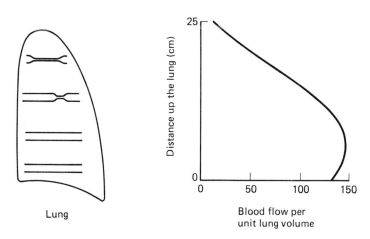

Lung

Blood flow per
unit lung volume

Fig. 6.3 Pulmonary blood flow in the erect human lung. Experiment performed using radioactive xenon which was injected intravenously and evolved into the alveolar gas on the first pass through the lung. The radioactivity of each region is proportional to the blood flow. (Redrawn, with permission, from J. M. B. Hughes et al., 1968, *Respiration Physiology*, **4**, 58–72.)

Distribution of blood in the lung

It was mentioned above that the blood flow is unevenly distributed in the lung of the resting upright human. This could result from purely passive factors imposed upon the circulation by its position in the thorax or from active control. Both are involved in the control of regional blood flow under different circumstances.

In the normal subject at sea level the uneven distribution of blood can be explained by local physical forces. Figure 6.3 shows the blood flow in the lung of a sitting human measured using isotopic techniques. The flow at the base of the lungs is high and at the apex very low. Because there is a column of blood 30 cm high, stretching from the base of the lungs to the apex, the hydrostatic pressure in the capillaries of the base of the lung will be higher than at the apex. The capillaries are surrounded by alveoli and the ambient pressure in the alveolar gas is usually close to atmospheric, so any pulmonary capillary in which the blood pressure falls to (or below) atmospheric will collapse. If the mean arterial blood pressure is 15 mmHg, the forward pressure in the capillaries at the apex of the lung 15 cm above the heart will be very small and flow will cease. The forward pressure at the base of the lung 10 cm below the heart will be closer to 30 mmHg and flow rapid. However, the blood flow cannot be predicted by consideration of the arterial pressure without reference to the pressures in the venous side of the circulation. Left atrial pressure averages 5 mmHg. The pressure in any pulmonary vein rising more than 5 cm above the left atrium will be atmospheric and will provide no resistance to pulmonary blood flow. It will also provide no distending pressure which would maintain the pulmonary capillary volume. The pulmonary veins draining the bases have a pressure greater than left atrial by the hydrostatic pressure imposed by the height of the column of blood within those veins. This provides a 'back' pressure of about 15 mmHg 10 cm below the left atrium, counteracting the forward pressure of the pulmonary artery, reducing flow and distending the pulmonary capillary bed. This simple consideration of pressures in the blood vessels leads to the conclusion that blood flow and capillary volume at the apex of the lung would be very low and would be maximal at the base of the lung. It also suggests that small rises in pulmonary venous pressure would lead to expansion of the capillary volume in the upper parts of the lung and that a small increase in pulmonary artery pressure would recruit the apical capillaries to the circulation.

This discussion has ignored the changes in intrapleural pressure which occur with each respiratory cycle and will alter the delicate balance between alveolar and capillary pressure. The zones of perfusion set out in Fig. 6.3 will alter constantly with the respiratory cycle and, to a smaller extent, with the cardiac cycle. Despite the obvious oversimplification, the principles set out above provide an adequate explanation of observed facts.

Active control of regional pulmonary blood flow can be imposed upon this system. The existence of this mechanism is necessary since perfusion must be matched to ventilation and not just dependent upon zonal distribution. The mechanism which dominates the control of pulmonary arteriolar tone is the partial pressure of oxygen in the terminal alveolar duct (P_{AO_2}). A fall in P_{AO_2} causes vasoconstriction in the accompanying pulmonary arteriole, reducing perfusion to the underventilated alveoli. Some lesser stimuli to vaso-constriction and vasodilation are listed in Table 6.1 but these will only alter the background tone upon which the local P_{AO_2} will act. The mechanism by which P_{AO_2} produces vasoconstriction is unknown, but it is crucial to matching perfusion to ventilation. When the inspired oxygen concentration falls, the same mechanism produces generalized vasoconstriction of the pulmonary arteries. Ascent to altitude produces generalized pulmonary

Table 6.1   Stimuli altering the pulmonary arteriolar tone

Increase tone ⟶ *Vasoconstriction*	*Decrease tone* ⟶ *Vasodilation*
Alveolar hypoxia:	Alveolar hypocapnia:
Alveolar hypercapnia	β-adrenergic agonists
α-adrenergic agonists	Prostaglandin E_1
Serotonin	Theophylline
Angiotensin II	
Prostaglandin $F_{2\alpha}$	

vasoconstriction and pulmonary hypertension. In normal humans this does no harm. In humans with diseased lungs it may lead to failure of the control of pulmonary blood flow at a local level, making the arterial hypoxaemia more severe by reducing the efficiency with which perfusion is matched to ventilation, or it may cause the right ventricle to hypertrophy and decompensate.

Other functions of the normal pulmonary circulation

Because the whole of the systemic venous return passes through the pulmonary capillary bed, the pulmonary circulation is ideally situated to act as a physical and a chemical filter. There is increasing evidence that these functions are important.

The role of the lung as a mechanical filter has long been recognized. Thrombus formation in the systemic venous system is common and pieces break off forming solid emboli in the venous return. The lung circulation has sufficient reserve capacity that more than 50 per cent of the vascular bed can be occluded with no rise in pulmonary artery pressure and small thrombotic pulmonary emboli lodge unnoticed. Once impacted, they are broken up by the pulsatile action of the blood and the fibrinolytic mechanisms. Complete restoration of the normal pulmonary blood flow is the outcome of all but the largest thrombotic pulmonary emboli (see below). This mechanical filtration protects the more vulnerable systemic circulation. When an abnormal connection exists between the right and left side of the heart, this filter is bypassed and the devastating effects of embolization of the systemic arterial tree are more commonly seen (e.g. cerebrovascular occlusion leading to brain damage or stroke). The filtration of the venous blood is also evident under other circumstances. When solid particles are inadvertently injected into the veins by doctors or are self-administered by drug addicts, the pulmonary circulation collects them. When infected particles are filtered, lung abscesses result. The high incidence of lung abscess in drug addicts illustrates the efficiency of the pulmonary filter. Another source of solid emboli is malignant tumours. When malignant tumours grow, they invade blood vessels and release clumps of cells into the venous blood stream. These are removed by the pulmonary capillary bed and are manifest by the pulmonary secondary deposits which are so commonly seen in disseminated malignant tumours. Fat droplets are released in extensive bony trauma and these can be such a large load to the pulmonary filter that extreme breathlessness and the expectoration of fat droplets in sputum occur.

For the same reasons that the lung is a good mechanical filter, it is ideally situated to alter the level of chemical substances reaching the systemic circulation. Just as the arterial oxygen and carbon dioxide content are determined by the action of the lung, humoral agents are inactivated, synthesized and released or converted in the pulmonary circulation. The pulmonary endothelium is rich in an enzyme called angiotensin-converting enzyme, and the relatively inactive angiotensin I is converted to angiotensin II in the pulmonary circulation. In this way the systemic circulation receives an active compound after passage through the pulmonary capillary bed. Angiotensin-coverting enzyme also degrades bradykinin, thereby protecting the systemic circulation from the vasodilating effect of the hormone. The prostaglandins provide further examples of these protective properties. Prostaglandins E_1 (vasodilator) and F_2 (vasoconstrictor) are inactivated in the pulmonary vascular bed, but prostacyclin (vasodilator) passes unchanged. Only prostacyclin causes systemic circulatory disturbance when given as intravenous infusion. Administered drugs may be bound by the pulmonary endothelium (propranolol) or metabolized (noradrenaline), altering the therapeutic effect. These are a few examples of the lung as a metabolic organ, and disruption of the normal lung can disturb these functions as well as the function of gas exchange.

Damaged lung

If the structure of the lung is damaged, function deteriorates. The effects of disease or damage of the different parts of the lung on pulmonary circulation are considered in turn.

Loss of lung tissue (e.g. pneumonectomy)

When lung tissue is lost following trauma or through operative resection, the remaining pulmonary circulation has to accept the total output of the right ventricle. Provided the remaining lung is normal, one of the two lungs can be removed without inducing symptoms (e.g. breathlessness) or significant change in function. There is no rise in the measured pulmonary artery pressure at rest. On exercise the reduced pulmonary capillary bed leads to a more rapid rise in pulmonary artery pressure with increasing cardiac output, but this does not limit the ability to perform moderate exercise.

If the whole blood volume is delivered to a smaller pulmonary capillary bed, the velocity of the blood in each capillary must be increased. This will reduce the time each red blood corpuscle spends in contact with the alveolar gas. However, gas exchange is so rapid that under normal circumstances the exchange of oxygen and carbon dioxide is completed within the first half of the pulmonary capillary (Widdicombe and Davies: *Respiratory Physiology*, Chapter 4). The efficiency of gas exchange is not reduced by the increased capillary blood velocity which follows the removal of one lung. The arterial

tensions of oxygen and carbon dioxide remain unchanged.
The mechanical filtration of the systemic venous blood and the metabolic function of the lung are not affected by pneumonectomy.
These statements assume that the structure and function of the remaining lung are normal. If only damaged lung remains, the loss of any lung tissue may lead to severely deranged function and to disabling symptoms. Some examples of how this may occur are discussed below.

Loss of peripheral lung tissue (e.g. emphysema)

The loss of alveolar tissue from the lung causes severe impairment of gas exchange, not only because the area for gas exchange is reduced but also because the loss of elasticity of the lung leads to other changes which reduce the efficient matching of perfusion and ventilation.

The loss of peripheral lung tissue reduces the pulmonary capillary network and the pulmonary capillary blood volume. For a given cardiac output the blood must travel faster through the remaining capillaries and this requires a higher pulmonary artery pressure. The more rapid flow means that the blood spends less time in contact with the alveolar air. Since the time taken for gas exchange is normally rapid, this will have little effect on arterial oxygenation in the resting subject. When the subject exercises and the cardiac output is raised then the rapidity of the flow through the reduced capillary bed may be so great as to limit gas exchange. These are the obvious effects of loss of alveolar tissue, but the damage does not end there.

The loss of elastic tissue in the lung allows the collapse of airways in expiration. This leads to an increase in resting lung volumes and in the intra-thoracic pressure swings of resting ventilation. The most dramatic change is a sharp increase in the expiratory intrathoracic pressure which may rise many centimetres above ambient atmospheric pressure. When the pressure in the alveolar air rises it causes compression of the pulmonary capillaries, further diminishing the pulmonary capillary bed. The high intrathoracic pressure also reduces systemic venous return and causes a sharp fall in right ventricular output. This causes a fall in pulmonary artery pressure and reduces the forward pressure for pulmonary blood flow. These effects may be so marked in severely emphysematous patients that right ventricular output and pulmonary blood flow virtually cease during expiration. This compounds the problem of rapid capillary blood flow because the whole cardiac output must traverse the reduced capillary bed during the inspiratory phase of the respiratory cycle, further decreasing the capillary transit time. When all these physiological disturbances are considered it is not surprising that the patient with extensive emphysema is severely disabled by breathlessness. The high lung volumes and large pressure swings induce vagal afferent discharge, leading to breathlessness at rest. To maintain airway patency in expiration the patient may exhale through pursed lips, thereby raising airways and intrathoracic pressure above ambient atmospheric. This has catastrophic effects on pulmonary blood flow during expiration, reducing cardiac output and adding to the physiological disturbance. The marked decrease in capillary transit time of the blood and poor matching of perfusion and ventilation lead to arterial hypoxaemia and exacerbate the sensation of breathlessness. When any exercise is attempted, the drive to breathe forces even larger intrathoracic pressure swings and leads rapidly to crippling breathlessness. Since lost alveolar tissue cannot be replaced, the prospect for the patient with severe emphysema is bleak.

None of the changes listed above interferes with the function of filtration of the venous blood, which remains intact. However, the metabolic functions of the pulmonary circulation depend upon the endothelial area to which the blood is exposed. Loss of peripheral lung tissue causes a marked loss of endothelium and severely limits the metabolic activity of the lung. In emphysema the inactivation of hormones and the absorption of drugs in the pulmonary circulation are reduced. It is possible that the passage of hormones normally inactivated by the lung into the systemic circulation contributes to the weight loss and breathlessness which mark this disease.

Disease producing patchy alveolar filling

In contrast to the emphysematous patient, the patient with oedema or infection of the alveoli has little loss of peripheral lung tissue. The function is temporarily disturbed, but the structure remains intact. Removal of the fluid from the alveoli will restore the lung to its normal state. Examples of this disturbance are oedema caused by high pulmonary venous pressure (transudate, described in Chapter 4), protein-rich oedema caused by leaky pulmonary capillaries (exudate: Chapter 4) and pneumonia or accumulation of cell-rich thick fluid.

Oedema induced by circulatory abnormalities
When the pulmonary venous pressure rises, pulmonary capillary pressure may exceed the osmotic pressure of the plasma proteins, forcing a transudate of plasma into the tissue space. Because pulmonary venous pressure is highest at the base of the lungs, the fluid accumulation is most severe in this region. When the tissue spaces are distended, lymphatic drainage increases but this may be overwhelmed and fluid allowed to spill into the alveolar spaces. This disrupts ventilation, reduces Pa_{O_2}, and perfusion to these areas of lung is reduced by the hypoxic vasoconstriction of the pulmonary arterioles. This redistributes the pulmonary blood flow to the apices of the lung, minimizing ventilation/perfusion mismatch and causes a rise in pulmonary artery pressure. If the pulmonary oedema is extensive, arterial hypoxaemia is severe, pulmonary hypertension is severe and the lungs become stiff. The patient with a myocardial infarct who is severely breathless, cyanosed and coughing frothy sputum is an extreme example of this problem. The pulmonary circulation remains intact but fails to maintain pulmonary blood flow or arterial oxygenation. If the left heart failure is treated and pulmonary venous pressure falls, the pulmonary oedema disappears and the patient returns to normal.

Oedema caused by leaky pulmonary capillaries
Oedema of the lung can occur with normal pulmonary arterial and pulmonary venous pressures if the integrity of the pulmonary capillary membrane is

breached. In severe infections, inhalation of toxic chemicals or after severe trauma the pulmonary endothelium can sustain damage, allowing protein-rich fluid to pour into the lung. This is known as the adult respiratory distress syndrome, and may require drastic measures such as positive pressure mechanical ventilation to maintain adequate gas exchange while the cause is treated. The disturbances to the pulmonary circulation are the same as with haemodynamic oedema (transudate), and treatment should achieve complete resolution.

Little is known about the metabolic function of the pulmonary endothelium in this condition. Since the primary abnormality is injury to the pulmonary endothelium, it would be surprising if it were not severely disturbed.

Infection of the lung (e.g. pneumonia)
In pneumonia the inflammatory reaction leads to the accumulation of protein-rich fluid and leucocytes in the infected area. If the primary site of the infection is the large airways (bronchopneumonia), patches of alveolar tissue around these bronchi become flooded. In the normal lung local pulmonary arterial constriction redirects the blood to unaffected areas of lung and there is no serious disruption of gas exchange. If the rest of the lung is abnormal then there may be no reserve areas to which blood can be redirected. This is the case in the chronic bronchitic who has generalized abnormalities of airways. When such a patient has an 'acute exacerbation' he may become severely ill with systemic hypoxaemia due to ventilation/perfusion mismatch. Physiotherapy to clear the bronchi will rapidly restore the ventilation to much of the lung and does more to help these patients than any other single therapeutic measure.

When one whole lobe of the lung is infected and flooded with inflammatory exudate, a similar sequence of events is triggered. This illness often occurs in fit people with normal lungs, and the regulation of the pulmonary circulation minimizes the disturbance to gas exchange by shutting off the blood supply to the infected lobe. This can be demonstrated in experimental animals and is seen in patients when the isotopic technique of lung scanning shows that an infected lobe has little perfusion and fails to ventilate. The redistribution of blood to normally ventilated areas occurs on the lobar scale as well as at the local level. Treatment of the pneumonia allows the lung to return to normal.

Diffuse patchy alveolar filling due to local damage (e.g. extrinsic allergic alveolitis or pneumoconiosis)
When local inflammatory reactions are caused by inhalation of antigen or by the inhalations of irritant dust, the areas of damage induced will be distributed according to the deposition of the particles in the airways. The resultant inflammatory exudation causes alveolar flooding in a widespread and patchy manner. The response of the pulmonary circulation to local airway hypoxia is vasoconstriction of the arterial tree proximal to the affected area. This is an inappropriate response to such patchy changes in the lung, since effective shunting of blood away from all affected areas induces generalized pulmonary vasoconstriction and a marked rise in pulmonary artery pressure, reducing blood flow to adjacent areas of unaffected lung. Modification of the

vasoconstriction to reduce these damaging consequences inevitably leads to perfusion of flooded alveoli and allows intrapulmonary shunting of systemic venous blood, causing arterial hypoxaemia. Subsequent fibrosis of the inflamed tissue perpetuates the abnormality and produces a sharp reduction in exercise tolerance and eventually breathlessness at rest.

Pulmonary arterial block (e.g. pulmonary embolism)

The filtration of solid particles from the mixed venous blood is a normal role of the pulmonary circulation. It is probably a regular event to have small thrombi or aggregations of platelets impacting in the pulmonary arterial tree, and the integrity of the pulmonary circulation depends upon its ability to remove the solid material and restore flow. Consideration of patients with pulmonary embolism, or the arrival of thrombus in the pulmonary arterial bed, will illustrate this property.

The way in which patients with pulmonary embolism present to the clinician depends upon the size of the thrombus. There are three distinct patterns of presentation.

1. The first is progressive breathlessness, without pain or coughing blood. This is the way in which many *small* emboli arriving over a long time will present. The pathological changes are occlusion of small patches of pulmonary capillaries without gross disturbance to regional blood flow or gas distribution. Over the years the thrombolytic and phagocytic mechanisms fail to clear all the thrombi and patchy permanent occlusions accumulate until the pulmonary vascular tree can no longer accommodate the right ventricular output. This leads to pulmonary arterial hypertension, right ventricular hypertrophy and peripheral oedema (swollen ankles). The scarred lungs become small and stiff, leading to breathlessness. These changes are permanent.

2. If a larger thrombus arrives, blocking a pulmonary artery such as the right main pulmonary artery, the consequences are different. This sudden catastrophic haemodynamic event leads to diversion of all the right ventricular output through the left lung, causing it to be congested and stiff. The right lung is ventilated but not perfused and reflex bronchoconstriction reduces its ventilation, stiffening this lung. Thus pulmonary blood flow and air flow are impaired, the lungs are stiffened and the output of the right side of the heart is impaired. This leads to the immediate symptoms of sudden breathlessness and wheeze. The subsequent progression of the pathological changes provides the basis for the other symptoms of haemoptysis (coughing blood) and pleuritic chest pain (sharp pain on breathing). In this example the bronchial circulation to the right lung remains intact. This allows the lung tissue to remain viable but provides a supply of blood which exudes into the alveolar spaces and is the source of the bloody sputum. The bloody alveolar exudate generates an inflammatory reaction in the affected lung, leading to pleuritic pain, a pleural rub and accumulation of a bloody pleural effusion. These are the symptoms and signs associated with a moderate sized pulmonary embolus.

The clinical picture which follows the initial deterioration is one of resolution and can be explained by the evolution of the pathological changes.

The pulsation of the pulmonary artery and the recruitment of fibrinolytic mechanisms break up the occluding thrombus. As the fragments move into the peripheral arteries the perfusion is restored to patches of the lung. This occurs over some hours and contributes to the observation that pulmonary emboli are multiple. The imperfect matching of perfusion and ventilation in the embolized pulmonary segment leads to perfused and underventilated segments, intrapulmonary shunting of venous blood and arterial hypoxaemia. The symptom of breathlessness resolves as the lung perfusion is restored.

Because the structure of the lung is preserved by the bronchial circulation, complete restoration of normal lung architecture can be expected.

3. The occlusion of the main pulmonary artery by an embolus leads to circulatory collapse and sudden death. Thrombi of this size usually originate from the large pelvic veins or the inferior vena cava. Rapid arrival of smaller emboli can lead to the same degree of circulatory collapse if the pulmonary defence mechanisms cannot clear previous emboli sufficiently fast.

Chronic hypoxia

Exposure to a reduced inspired oxygen tension
The response of the pulmonary circulation to a low inspired oxygen tension is generalized vasoconstriction. When humans are exposed to a low inspired P_{O_2}, either by reducing the fraction of oxygen in the inspired air or by ascending to altitude, the pulmonary artery pressure rises. The rise in pulmonary artery pressure is greater the lower the inspired P_{O_2}. Because the fall in arterial Pa_{O_2} leads to an increase in minute ventilation and the rise in pulmonary arterial pressure increases the perfusion of the lung apices, ventilation and perfusion remain matched. This makes best use of the limited supply of oxygen. Later changes induced by hypoxia, such as polycythaemia, may improve blood oxygen-carrying capacity but will increase the pulmonary artery pressure still further as the blood viscosity rises. This does not cause any reduction in pulmonary vasoconstriction and increases right ventricular work. On prolonged exposure to hypoxia histological changes occur in the small pulmonary arteries, leading to increased thickness of the muscle coat, an extra elastic lamina and narrowing of the lumen. Once established, these changes take many months to resolve when the inspired oxygen tension rises. On return to sea level the pulmonary artery pressure of high altitude dwellers shows only a small fall initially and then a gradual decline to normal levels over the succeeding months. The initial fall represents relaxation of active vasoconstriction and the slow decline the regression of hypertrophy of small pulmonary arteries.

Arterial hypoxia caused by underventilation or abnormal lungs
Whatever the cause of arterial hypoxaemia, the pulmonary circulation responds by constriction of the small arteries. As discussed above, this evens the perfusion to normal lungs and enables the extraction of oxygen from the alveolar air to be as efficient as possible. When arterial hypoxia is caused by underventilation, this is an appropriate response.

In an abnormal lung arterial hypoxaemia is limited by reducing the pulmonary blood flow to the underventilated areas. Generalized pulmonary vasoconstriction destroys the regional control of blood flow and reduces the proportion of the pulmonary blood flow selectively directed to the ventilated areas. This increases the shunting of blood across the pulmonary circulation and allows arterial P_{O_2} to decline. In this instance the hypoxic vasoconstrictor response is inappropriate, causing a deterioration of the arterial P_{O_2}—the variable it normally protects. The only way to break this damaging circle of cause and effect is to improve alveolar ventilation. This allows arterial P_{O_2} to rise and pulmonary arterial pressure to fall, in turn allowing a greater degree of regional control of blood flow.

These principles are illustrated by the chronic bronchitic with an acute exacerbation. The acute infection increases the production of mucus secretions and blocks airways. The blocked airways allow segmental collapse of lung and produce arterial hypoxaemia through the perfusion of unventilated lung. The immediate treatment is to clear the airways and restore ventilation. This is achieved by chest physiotherapy. Antibiotics treat the infection and reduce production of mucus but do not restore ventilation unless the accumulated sputum is expectorated. Severe arterial hypoxaemia with consequent pulmonary hypertension is avoided by maintaining ventilation and the patient recovers more rapidly. Increasing the inspired P_{O_2} by oxygen administration may do little to improve arterial P_{O_2} unless the ventilation/perfusion mismatch is corrected. An oxygen mask is no substitute for physiotherapy in the treatment of exacerbations of chronic bronchitis.

Diseases posing peculiar problems for the pulmonary circulation

Congenital heart disease with left-to-right shunt of blood
In an atrial septal defect, a ventricular septal defect or a patent ductus arteriosus the blood flows from the systemic to the pulmonary circulation, as the pressures in the left side of the circulation are higher. Some of the pulmonary venous return is shunted back into the lungs via the pulmonary artery, loading the pulmonary circulation. The problem is to accommodate the increased blood flow without compromising the regulation of blood flow to ventilation in the lung.

Shunts of more than 50 per cent of pulmonary venous return can be accommodated when the lung is young and healthy, but eventually very high pulmonary blood flow leads to thickening of the pulmonary vessel walls, increased pulmonary artery pressure and reversal of the shunt. When this happens the pulmonary circulation is non-compliant, regulates regional flow poorly and the right-to-left shunting of blood destroys the integrity of the mechanical filtration and metabolic protective functions of the lung. This situation exists from birth in such conditions as Fallot's tetralogy (pulmonary stenosis and the ventricular septal defect), single ventricle or transposition of the great vessels. All of these impose severe limitations on the individual who is centrally cyanosed and has a shortened life expectancy.

Mitral stenosis
In mitral stenosis the valve between the left atrium and left ventricle is narrowed. This leads to a high left atrial pressure and pulmonary hypertension, especially during exercise when the cardiac output rises. When the pressure in the pulmonary veins is raised, the Starling equilibrium is disturbed and tissue fluid increases. This stiffens the lungs and causes breathlessness with a dry non-productive cough. The raised pulmonary venous pressure necessitates a higher pulmonary arterial pressure to maintain blood flow through the lung and increases pulmonary capillary blood volume. If pressures in the pulmonary vein are very high (2.7–4 kPa, 20-30 mmHg) then blood elements are forced into the interstitial spaces of the lung. When red blood cells are repeatedly extruded from the circulation and destroyed by pulmonary macrophages, local deposition of iron and fibrosis occurs. This condition is called pulmonary haemosiderosis and causes permanent stiffening of the lung and redistribution of blood flow.

If the valve abnormality is corrected in the early stages, when the lung is structurally intact, the symptoms resolve. In advanced mitral stenosis, when the lungs have developed pulmonary haemosiderosis, breathlessness is unremitting and does not resolve with haemodynamic correction.

Pulmonary changes in chronic liver disease
In certain forms of liver disease, particularly primary biliary cirrhosis, the lung develops multiple arteriovenous shunts. These can become so numerous that they produce a significant shunt of desaturated blood into the pulmonary veins, leading to systemic hypoxaemia. It also bypasses the metabolic activity of the pulmonary capillary endothelium, but the consequences of this are unknown.

7

Respiratory infections

The physiological impact of an infection of the respiratory tract will depend upon the infecting organism, the site of infection, the state of the whole patient and of the respiratory tract prior to the infection. The balance of these three variables determines the physiological changes which add up to the recognizable disease produced by the infection. Just as any infection of the bladder will produce painful and frequent micturition, infections of the larynx or the lung tissue produce recognizable collections of symptoms and signs irrespective of the nature of the causative organism. However, organisms can produce different diseases by infection of different sites, patients of different ages or patients with altered immunity. *Streptococcus pneumoniae* causes pneumonia when it infects the lung parenchyma of a healthy individual and an acute exacerbation in the bronchi of the chronic bronchitic. *Haemophilus influenzae* causes an exacerbation in the chronic bronchitic and acute epiglottitis in children. Cytomegalovirus causes enlarged lymph nodes, liver and spleen in normal individuals and confluent pneumonia in the immuno-suppressed patient. This interaction of organism, site of infection and the underlying state of the individual makes prediction of the physiological consequences of respiratory tract infections difficult. In this chapter are outlined the defences of the respiratory tract, with descriptions of the physiological changes expected from infections involving the extrathoracic airways (nose, throat, larynx), the large intrathoracic airways (trachea, bronchi) and the lung parenchyma followed by a scheme of management of the consequences of the altered physiology.

Defences of the normal respiratory tract

The lung is usually infected by inhalation of airborne organisms. The defences employed to prevent the organisms from establishing themselves in the airways or lungs are summarized in Table 7.1. They comprise the filtration of the inspired air, impaction and clearance before mucosal penetration is achieved, and tissue defences. Once tissue defences are mobilized, an inflammatory response is inevitable. The physiological consequences of respiratory infections depend upon the site and the extent of the inflammatory response.

Table 7.1   Defence mechanisms of the respiratory tract

Filtration of the air

Large particles (> 10 μm)
 Nasal hairs
 Impaction of droplets in turbulent flow or when air flow direction changes (e.g. posterior nasopharynx)

Small particles (< 0.1 μm)
 Remain suspended and are exhaled

Clearance of impacted particles

Continuous clearance of surface mucus – ciliary transport
Intermittent clearance – cough

Neutralization of specific antigens

Secreted IgA in surface mucus

Tissue defence mechanisms (in bronchial mucosa or alveolar tissue)

Humoral
 Immunoglobulins IgM, IgG
 (+ polymorphonuclear leucocyte)

Cellular
 Macrophage
 Lymphocyte

Effects on the whole body

The general effect of the acute inflammatory response of respiratory infections depends more upon the site and extent of the infection than upon the infecting organism. When the infection is confined to the conducting airways, the surface area of the inflammation is small and systemic symptoms of fever and malaise are less troublesome than cough and local pain. When the lung parenchyma is infected, the inflammatory response causes severe systemic upset. The characteristic manifestations of the pneumonia differ with each infecting organism (lobar pneumonia with *S. pneumoniae*, atypical pneumonia with *Mycoplasma pneumoniae*, Legionnaire's disease with *Legionella pneumophila*) but these clinical entities overlap and the clinical picture cannot be used to predict the infecting agent with accuracy.

Infections of the upper respiratory tract

Nasal air passages

When the nasal mucosa is infected, it swells and produces copious thin mucus. Because the nasal air passages are surrounded by bone, any swelling of the mucosa encroaches on the lumen and may occlude it. The secretions pour from the external nares or into the posterior nasopharynx, further embarrassing air flow and irritating the pharyngeal mucous membrane. The main effect of this is to increase airways resistance when the mouth is closed. In the adult human there is an automatic switch to continuous mouth-breathing which completely bypasses the obstruction. The residual physiological changes are consequent on the loss of normal nasal function, and comprise decreased efficiency of the humidification and warming of the inspired air. This is not serious at rest, but if minute ventilation is increased by exercising in a dry atmosphere, considerable cooling of the large airways occurs. This leads to irritant receptor discharge (cough) and may trigger bronchoconstriction, leading in turn to an attack of 'asthma'. Other than the discomfort of a 'cold', the physiological consequences are negligible.

Pharyngeal wall, larynx and related structures

Acute pharyngitis is uncomfortable and, if combined with tonsillitis, may cause high fever and severe systemic upset. There are no consequences to gas exchange or airways function if the epiglottis and larynx are spared.

In contrast, acute epiglottitis (which occurs most frequently in young children) or acute laryngitis may be life-threatening conditions because the airway may become completely obstructed. The epiglottis is situated behind the tongue and above the larynx, and if it swells it is in a position to occlude the laryngeal airway. Swelling of the vocal cords or false vocal cords can lead to restriction of the laryngeal lumen. Unfortunately, the onset of swelling in acute epiglottitis is rapid and upper airways resistance rises rapidly. This leads to increased inspiratory and expiratory effort, forcing air past the obstruction. Turbulent air flow leads to noisy breathing and an ineffective cough. Impaction of secretions may precipitate complete air flow obstruction and death. Since the infecting organism may be *H. influenzae*, which is easily treated with broad-spectrum antibiotics, this is a catastrophe because prompt recognition and treatment would allow the airway to return to normal. In this example, inflammation of the upper airways alters airway calibre so greatly that air flow is reduced below levels sufficient to maintain gas exchange. The dramatic physiological effect is produced by the position of the inflamed organ, not the extent of the infection.

The effect of chronic infections of the air sinuses, middle ear or nasal passages on pulmonary function is small.

Infections of the lower respiratory tract

These are most conveniently divided by their site into those occurring in the tubes and those occurring in the alveolar tissue.

Trachea and large bronchi

Acute and chronic infections of these large airways produce different clinical pictures and will be considered separately.

Acute tracheobronchitis
The acute inflammatory reaction to viral colonization of the trachea and large bronchi or of the bacterial invasion which may follow viral destruction of the

lining epithelium has effects on air flow and on gas exchange. The inflammatory process itself causes mucosal swelling and copious secretion of mucus. Either of these can block airways and cut the air supply to segments of lung, allowing their collapse and de-aeration (atelectasis). This alters the matching of ventilation to perfusion, causing inefficient gas exchange. It is most frequently seen in the dependent lower lobes. The second important effect of acute tracheobronchitis is that it denudes the epithelium, destroying the normal ciliated columnar pattern, disrupting mucus transport, altering the characteristics of the mucus (including the content of immunoglobulin IgA). This reduces the efficiency of mucus clearance, further impairing defence mechanisms. The exposure of the sensory nerve endings to the tidal air leads to cough and to bronchoconstriction. This can be demonstrated by challenging the airways with inhaled histamine. Bronchoconstriction can be produced with a much lower dose of histamine in the asthmatic or in the patient recovering from influenza than in the normal individual. The increased sensitivity of the airways to irritants can be demonstrated for up to 6 weeks after the infection, suggesting that the regeneration and reorganization of the mucous membrane is a lengthy process and that lung defences may be impaired long after the illness is over. The severe substernal pain on deep breathing or coughing typical of tracheitis is caused by excessive afferent vagal discharge and is the principal symptom of this infection.

A single attack of acute tracheobronchitis rarely leads to permanent structural damage. However, in certain circumstances permanent changes can take place. If the alveolar tissue around the bronchi becomes involved, a bronchopneumonia and patchy destruction of lung can occur (see below). If the regional lymph nodes swell during the infection, they can press on a bronchus from without and can narrow it. This is particularly important when the hilar lymph nodes constrict the orifice of a lobar bronchus, and can lead to poor ventilation and repeated episodes of infection in that lobe. However, both these represent extensions of the infection beyond the airways themselves.

Chronic bronchitis
Repeated infections of the large airways usually occur when the normal defence mechanisms have been weakened by the inhalation of irritant vapours or dusts over many years. The commonest cause of this is smoking, but living in a polluted atmosphere (e.g. the smoky atmosphere of London in the 1940s and 1950s before the Clean Air Act, or exposure at work as with blast furnace workers) can lead to the same structural changes. Pathologically, the bronchial mucosa becomes thicker, contains more mucus-secreting goblet cells and loses its cilia, the bronchial glands enlarge and the muscle wall hypertrophies (see Chapter 3). All of these changes encroach upon the lumen of the bronchi. The quality of the mucus secretion changes and it becomes loaded with migrating leucocytes. These changes lead to the patient noticing wheezy breathing due to the narrow tubes and cough productive of green or yellow sputum due to the increased mucus secretion and lack of mucociliary transport.

The pooling of excess secretions in the bronchi provides an ideal incubation medium for any infecting agent carried into the lung in the inspired air. When an organism infects the secretions in the bronchial tree, the changes induced by the organism and by the proteins released by lysed leucocytes cause increased mucus production and leucocyte migration. Copious quantities of dilute mucus are poured into the bronchi and expectorated. Unfortunately, the act of coughing involves a deep inspiration prior to the explosive expiration, and the secretions are thus sucked into the periphery of the lung. There the inhaled infected secretions lodge in the dependent small bronchi, blocking the tubes and causing segmental collapse and infection in the peripheral lung (bronchopneumonia) whilst the thin purulent secretions in the air tubes cause bronchial irritation and airways narrowing. This leads to the systemic symptoms of malaise and fever, and the physiological problems of air flow obstruction and of alveolar infection described below. Thus chronic bronchitis predisposes to bronchopneumonia, and repeated attacks lead to fibrosis and destruction of the affected segments in the dependent lower lobes.

Infections of the small air passages

Primary infection of the small air passages is common in children, and leads to severe abnormalities of air flow and of gas exchange. The clinical name of bronchiolitis is given to infections which are usually viral (respiratory syncytial virus or parainfluenza virus) and attack the peripheral small airways, causing swelling of the walls, occlusion of the lumen and local cessation of air flow. Because this is a patchy process occurring in all parts of the periphery of the lung, the effects are more similar to an alveolar infection (pneumonia) than an air-tube infection. The inflammatory process is too far down the bronchial tree to produce sputum, but involves the surrounding alveoli, producing patchy alveolar oedema, stiffening of the lung and severe systemic upset with fever and malaise. The patient complains of an irritating but non-productive or dry cough. The many patches of alveolar filling and local collapse interfere with gas exchange and may lead to severe hypoxaemia due to pulmonary shunting of venous blood. This causes breathlessness. In children the infection usually resolves with little permanent impairment of lung function. When this occurs in adults it frequently leads to permanent disability manifest by breathlessness and non-productive cough. Lung function tests show air flow obstruction with air-trapping and arterial desaturation.

Infections of the peripheral lung tissue

When an infection affects the alveolar tissue it is called a pneumonia. The most common pneumonic infection in normal people is caused by *Streptococcus pneumoniae* and is called lobar pneumonia. This is an illness which displays all the characteristics of acute infection of the alveoli, and a description of the clinical presentation will illustrate the physiological changes. A fit young man experiences a sudden severe pain in the right side of the chest. The pain is worse on breathing in and is accompanied by breathlessness and a cough. The pain is caused by inflammation of the visceral pleura (pleuritic pain) and the breathlessness by stiffening of the lung with widespread alveolar filling. The exudate spills from the infected lung, triggering vagal reflexes and causing cough which leads to worsening of the chest pain. These local effects are accompanied by severe prostration and high fever—the result of the products of inflammation flooding across the alveolar membrane into the capillary blood and their distribution in the systemic circulation. The damaged capillary membrane allows plasma and blood cells into the alveolar space and this bloody exudate is expectorated as thick red sputum. The alveolar filling leads to ventilation/perfusion mismatch and arterial hypoxaemia. There is no airways obstruction. Either the patient is overwhelmed by the infection and by penetration of bacteria into the systemic circulation (60 per cent of cases of lobar pneumonia have *S. pneumoniae* recovered from blood culture) or treatment and the immune mechanisms overcome the infection, leading to recovery. Because the structure of the lung is preserved, complete resolution is possible.

The complications of lobar pneumonia may cause permanent changes. The pleurisy indicates pleural inflammation, and an accumulation of pleural fluid may occur. If this contains bacteria, it attracts leucocytes into the pleural space and becomes an empyema. This leads to pleural fibrosis and splinting of the lung by encasement. If lysis of the fibrous skeleton of the lung ensues, a lung abscess develops. On recovery, this becomes a shrunken scar. Neither of these complications is serious, but they do restrict the measured total lung capacity.

Other causes of alveolar infection provide variations on this patern. The clinical picture of atypical pneumonia (*Mycoplasma pneumoniae*), Legionnaire's disease (*Legionella pneumophila*) and tuberculosis (*Mycobacterium tuberculosis*) are examples of the variation in clinical presentation which is seen in infections of the lung parenchyma. (Tuberculosis is discussed further in Chapter 9).

If the lungs are abnormal, the clinical features of the infection change. Stenosis of a major bronchus delays the clearing of secretions and repeated infections occur. This is often an early sign of carcinoma of the bronchus, and repeated infections of the same part of the lung which clear slowly should always raise this suspicion. The physiological disturbance is caused by the infection and following effective treatment there may be no detectable abnormality.

Similarly, the presence of a cavity within the lung or pleural space invites infection by a variety of normally non-pathogenic organisms (e.g. *Aspergillus fumigatus* in a tuberculous cavity). The symptoms and signs result from inflammation of the cavity wall and resolve with eradication of the infecting organism.

Clinical management of pneumonia

In an ideal world the clinician would be able to treat a respiratory infection knowing the organism involved and its antibiotic sensitivity. The preceding paragraphs have illustrated that this world is far from ideal. The clinical manifestations of an infection depend upon the host and the site of infection as well as the infecting organism. Without bacterial culture only an educated guess as to the organism and its sensitivity to treatment is possible. Most

Table 7.2 Initial management of pneumonia depending upon the clinical presentation

Clinical situation	Usual pathogen	Proposed treatment
A previously healthy person Contracted outside hospital	*Streptococcus pneumoniae*	Penicillin
Complication of viral illness	*Str. pneumoniae* *Staphylococcus aureus*	Penicillin + flucloxacillin
Pre-existing chronic bronchitis	*Str. pneumoniae* *Haemophilus influenzae*	Amoxycillin
Immunocompromised host (leukaemia, lymphoma or immunosuppressive therapy)	Common pathogens and many opportunistic organisms	Gentamicin + amoxycillin i.v. (obtain firm diagnosis)
Lung abscess	Gut organisms (the result of bloodborne infection or of aspiration)	Gentamicin, amoxycillin + metronidazole i.v.
Pneumonia distal to bronchial stenosis	*Str. pneumoniae* *Staph. aureus*	Penicillin or amoxycillin Flucloxacillin

cultures take 24–48 hours and some 6 weeks (*Mycobacterium tuberculosis*), so treatment must be started before the organism is identified. In Table 7.2 is proposed a practical scheme which takes into account the principles we have outlined and a knowledge of the common bacterial pathogens. All patients require supportive measures (advice about bed rest, diet and general nursing measures). In addition to the initial drug management outlined, the severe pneumonia may require physiotherapy and supplementary oxygen—both of which are best provided in hospital. When the pathogen is identified, the treatment may be modified to ensure the best chance of rapid resolution with minimum lung damage.

In the patient with abnormal immune responses normally non-pathogenic bacteria, viruses or protozoa can cause pneumonia or invade the blood stream. This complicates the treatment of lung infections in these patients because the usually recommended treatment takes no account of these unusual organisms. The frequency and severity of lung infections in the immuno-compromised patient is reflected by the high mortality from pneumonia. Early treatment with broad-spectrum antibiotics is mandatory; lung biopsy is often the only way to identify the infecting organism and is strongly recommended. This policy has greatly reduced the mortality from pneumonia in such patients.

Another special circumstance is the patient suffering from mucoviscidosis or cystic fibrosis. The abnormally tenacious mucus of such patients is usually colonized by *Staphylococcus aureus* or *Pseudomonas aeruginosa*. Early treatment of chest infections with antibiotics active against these organisms and repeated chest physiotherapy is necessary to allow recovery with the minimum of lung damage.

8

Acid-base disorders

This chapter concerns an important aspect of respiration—that is, its contribution to acid-base control. This is important because respiration becomes linked with all the other mechanisms which contribute to the stability of pH in the body (Table 8.1). Any 'final solution' of an acid-base disorder must depend on adjustment of the respiratory excretion of CO_2 or of the urinary pH. (The principles involved in acid-base control have been reviewed in Widdicombe and Davies: *Respiratory Physiology*, Chapter 5.) This chapter presents a clinical approach founded on those facts which seem helpful in dealing with acid-base disorders.

Table 8.1 Mechanisms contributing to the control of body pH

Buffering mechanisms:
Haemoglobin
CO_2-H_2CO_3
Proteins
Phosphates
Respiratory excretion of CO_2
Renal adjustment of urinary pH.

Once acid-base disorders are considered in a clinical context we are concerned with two aspects: first, the analysis of the abnormality (diagnosis); and second, (when appropriate) treatment. In order to understand acid-base problems we must go far outside the bounds of respiration, and for this reason the chapter starts with a brief outline of the factors which will be important (this should be viewed as a supplement to Widdicombe and Davies: *Respiratory Physiology*, Chapter 5).

Basics of the control of body pH

The processes which control body pH are listed in Table 8.1. The efficiency of these mechanisms is demonstrated in a classic experiment described by Pitts in

1953; intravenous infusion of hydrochloric acid into a dog produced a fall in arterial pH from 7.44 to 7.18, a dangerous but not lethal level of acidaemia. Addition of the same volume of acid to a volume of water approximating the total body water of the dog reduced the pH to 1.8. Basically, this chapter is concerned with the processes which limited the fall in pH in the dog.

Buffering mechanisms within the body

These constitute an immediate mechanism for dealing with acid–base disorders because they are instantly available to limit the change of pH. The most important, quantitatively, of these buffers is haemoglobin.

The reaction

$$H^+ + Hb^- \rightleftharpoons HHb$$

will minimize the change in blood pH whether the increase in the number of hydrogen ions (H^+) is brought about by the addition of acids to the body fluids or by the transport of CO_2 from tissues to the lungs for excretion. In the latter case, haemoglobin is remarkably well adapted for this purpose because its buffering power changes with reduction and oxygenation. Reduced haemoglobin is a stronger base (it can bind more H^+) than oxygenated haemoglobin. This enables the haemoglobin which has surrendered its O_2 in the capillaries to carry more H^+ away from the tissues where they have been produced. Haemoglobin is an intracellular buffer and its value depends on the ease with which CO_2 diffuses into red cells; it contributes a highly specialized buffering mechanism for the special requirements of blood. The role of intracellular buffering in general is considered later in this chapter.

Fundamental to acid-base physiology is the hydration of CO_2 to form carbonic acid and the dissociation of the acid:

$$CO_2 + H_2O \rightleftharpoons H_2CO_3 \rightleftharpoons H^+ + HCO_3^-$$

This reaction is of importance because it relates the respiratory excretion of CO_2 to acid–base balance. An increase in the number of H^+ on the right side of the equation will displace the reaction to the left, increasing the CO_2 available to the lungs for exhalation. The mechanisms listed in Table 8.1 as contributing to buffering are all, with the exception of haemoglobin, extracellular. Is there any contribution from the intracellular compartment (other than red blood cells) to the buffering mechanisms? This topic is central to the subject of pH control, and the exchanges which occur between intracellular fluid (ICF) and extracellular fluid (ECF) in acid–base disorders are fundamental to the understanding of clinical acid–base problems. Acid-base disorders rarely exist on their own and are usually associated with abnormalities in the distribution of H_2O, Na^+ and K^+, which may be clinically more important than the changes in blood pH.

Role of intracellular–extracellular exchanges

Again, the classic experiment of Pitts can be used as a starting point. Infusion of hydrochloric acid into a dog produced a severe extracellular acidosis; in the time of the experiment renal mechanisms would have made a negligible contribution. The acid load was dealt with entirely by available buffers and respiratory excretion of CO_2. To what extent were the buffering mechanisms entirely confined to the ECF or were intracellular mechanisms involved? In a careful balance calculation 30–50 per cent of the acid load was buffered within cells. In addition, there was an exchange of Na^+ and K^+, both ions leaving cells and entering the ECF. In a similar experiment with a sodium bicarbonate load, approximately 30 per cent of the load was accounted for intracellularly. Clearly pH control is not brought about by solely extracellular mechanisms, yet most of our calculations are based on, and directed towards consideration of, purely extracellular mechanisms. This attitude is determined by our considerable ignorance of intracellular pH (pHi) and its control. In any discussion of acid–base disorders, changes in pHi must be of importance because it is intracellular mechanisms which will determine the metabolic response to such a disorder.

Intracellular pH

The measurement of pHi is a research technique and there is little information available from diseased man. Certain facts about pHi are established and these carry important implications. First, cells are more acid than the ECF. At a pH of 7.4 in the ECF, cellular pH is about 7.0. Even this basic finding has been subject to controversy. Considerable doubts have existed concerning the methods used, the inhomogeneity of the intracellular fluid and the differences which must exist between cells from different tissues. In spite of these doubts, a value for pHi around 7.0 seems acceptable and, if this is so, we must accept from this an important implication. If extracellular pH (pHe) is 7.4 and most cells support an electrical potential across the cell membrane, the inside of the cell being approximately 60 mV negative to the exterior then we can calculate that the hydrogen ion (H^+) is out of electrochemical equilibrium. If it were passively distributed, pHi would be about 6.0. Even if there are doubts concerning the measurement of pHi, we can be sufficiently confident about the figure of 7.0 to be convinced that H^+ is out of electrochemical equilibrium. The most likely explanation is that H^+ is actively extruded from the cell against this electrochemical gradient. Recent work using pHi-sensitive electrodes has produced evidence for such an active extrusion of H^+. If, therefore, cells are permeable to H^+ (see experiments of Pitts described above) and H^+ can be actively extruded from cells then the role of the intracellular contribution in any acid–base derangement will be complicated. A detailed consideration of pHi control is not appropriate here. Intracellular pH control can be related to three mechanisms:

1. Physicochemical buffering within cells; intracellular proteins will, for example, contribute to this.
2. The consumption or production by the cell of organic acids (e.g. lactate).
3. Transmembrane fluxes of H^+; an active extrusion of H^+ as described above is probably implicated.

Perhaps it is appropriate at this point to consider the implications of this to clinical problems. In the Pitts experiment infusion of an acid produced a fall in pHe, H^+ entered cells, and Na^+ and K^+ left cells to pass into the ECF. This establishes that abnormalities in H^+ distribution cannot be considered on their own for they will be associated with changes in the distribution of other ions. These exchanges may well be complicated. For example, in an acidosis K^+ leaves liver and skeletal muscle whereas it appears to enter cardiac muscle. We must be careful, therefore, not to extrapolate from the behaviour of one tissue to that of another. The infusion of an acid intravenously is an experimental simplification because in disease states the acid will be generated intra-cellularly in most circumstances, and the acids will then diffuse from the affected tissues into the ECF and thence into other less affected tissues.

The lessons to be learnt from this discussion are:

1. Measurements of pHe may not always tell us very much about pHi.
2. pHi and its relation to movement of K^+ may vary from tissue to tissue.

In view of the latter point, attempts to investigate pHi in disease states by examination of a biopsy specimen (usually skeletal muscle) may not be of value in predicting events in other more crucial tissues such as heart. An example of the problem comes from severe potassium depletion. Hypo-kalaemia is associated under these conditions with an ECF alkalosis. This may be accounted for rather simply by the assumption that K^+ has left some cells to be replaced by H^+ and Na^+. This is certainly true in skeletal muscle, since an intracellular acidosis can be shown to develop. This emphasizes the point that in some circumstances pHi and pHe may be dissociated, for an ECF alkalosis is associated with an intracellular acidosis in skeletal muscle. Measurement of pHe alone might be misleading. Similarly, it is not justified to extrapolate from one tissue to another. Although K^+ depletion leads to loss of K^+ from skeletal muscle and the development of an intracellular acidosis, this does not occur in cardiac muscle which does not lose K^+ nor does pHi change. Since we have little information as yet concerning changes in pHi, this must remain a confused field. It serves to emphasize, though, that ECF acid–base analysis can at best be only a guide to intracellular events and that disorders of H^+ distribution will be accompanied by significant shifts of Na^+ and K^+ between ECF and ICF.

These considerations provide the background against which we must consider methods of analysing acid–base disorders and finally how to treat them.

An approach to the analysis of acid-base problems based on clinical observation

Simple problems

Very often, acid–base physiology seems to be concerned solely with artificial problems divorced from clinical circumstances. The techniques of acid–base analysis should be used to confirm a clinical diagnosis and to quantify the abnormality. The diagnosis of diabetic ketoacidosis is seldom reached via acid–base measurements but, having made the diagnosis, acid–base measurements are necessary to quantify the severity of the acidaemia. It will be assumed that the readers of this chapter have started by examining the patient, that a diagnosis has been reached and that acid–base analysis will be used to confirm the decision. Table 8.2 indicates some of the common causes of alkalosis and acidosis related to the fundamental reaction of acid–base physiology, namely the hydration of CO_2. The analysis of an acid–base

Table 8.2 Some common causes of acidosis and alkalosis

$$CO_2 + H_2O \rightleftharpoons H_2CO_3 \rightleftharpoons H^+ + HCO_3$$

Respiratory		Metabolic	
alkalosis	acidosis	alkalosis	acidosis
Pregnancy	Airways obstruction	K^+ loss:	Diabetic ketoacidosis
Hypoxia	Neuromuscular disorders	Vomiting	Renal failure
Anxiety	Brain damage	Diuretics	Lactic acidosis:
Hysteria	Drug overdose:	Conn's syndrome	Diabetes
Artificial ventilation	Barbiturates	Cushing's syndrome	Tissue hypoxia
Salicylate overdose (adults)	Opiates	Laxatives	Phenformin
		Acid loss:	Septicaemia
		Vomiting	Renal tubular acidosis
		Pyloric stenosis	
		Gastric aspiration	
		Alkali infusion (or ingestion)	

problem is easier nowadays because the appropriate measurements are in routine clinical use. For most simple situations the measurement of the pH and $P\text{CO}_2$ of arterial blood are sufficient. The former is a direct measurement of any deviation from the normal range of arterial pH (7.35–7.45) and the latter a direct measurement of the respiratory component. To be correct, any process which tends to acidify or alkalinize blood but which does not alter pH outside these limits should be called an acidosis or alkalosis. When the control of pH fails to contain the process within these limits, it is an acidaemia or an alkalaemia. An arterial $P\text{CO}_2$ within the normal limits (4.7–6 kPa, 35–45 mmHg) indicates that alveolar ventilation is appropriate for that CO_2 production, a low $P\text{CO}_2$ indicating excessive ventilation and a high $P\text{CO}_2$-deficient alveolar ventilation. Table 8.3 shows that most simple acute acid-base problems can be solved by a measurement of pH and $P\text{CO}_2$. Every acid-base problem can be analysed in terms of two components: the initial event which led to the disturbance, and the compensatory reaction which will minimize the change in pH. If, for example, ventilation fails, the arterial $P\text{CO}_2$

Table 8.3   Arterial pH, P_{CO_2} and $[HCO_3^-]$ in simple acid-base disorders

	Arterial		
	pH	P_{CO_2}	$[HCO_3^-]$
Acidosis:			
Respiratory	↓	**↑**	↑
Metabolic	**↓**	↓	↓
Alkalosis:			
Respiratory	↑	**↓**	↓
Metabolic	**↑**	↑	↑

Bold arrow indicates primary change

will rise, producing a respiratory acidosis. Initially, the fall in arterial pH is limited by the available extracellular and intracellular buffers. Final compensation must come from an adjustment of the renal excretion of H^+ and HCO_3^-. This adjustment in renal excretion will bring about an increase in plasma $[HCO_3^-]$ and a consequent return of arterial pH towards normal. The primary abnormality, a respiratory acidosis, is compensated for by a secondary metabolic alkalosis. Before compensation is complete, acute acid-base problems are usually easy to solve. At this stage, pH and P_{CO_2} are the discriminating measurements. Before electrodes which measured pH and P_{CO_2} directly became generally available, plasma $[HCO_3^-]$ or some related measurement made even acute changes a confusing topic. As Table 8.3 shows, $[HCO_3^-]$ is not a discriminating variable, for it will move in the same direction both in a respiratory acidosis and in a metabolic alkalosis. The fundamental variables of acid-base analysis are related by the central reaction:

$$H_2O + CO_2 \rightleftharpoons H_2CO_3 \rightleftharpoons H^+ + HCO_3^-$$

The right-hand part of the equation can be conveniently rearranged using the law of mass action:

$$\frac{[H^+]\,[HCO_3^-]}{[CO_2]} = K$$

Note: $[CO_2]$ is written for H_2CO_3 because $[H_2CO_3]$ is proportional to the concentration of dissolved CO_2.

By changing this into a logarithmic form (giving pH and pK) and rearranging we obtain:

$$pH = pK + \log \frac{[HCO_3^-]}{[CO_2]}$$

Finally, since dissolved CO_2 is proportional to the P_{CO_2}, we can substitute αP_{CO_2} for $[CO_2]$ where α is the solubility of CO_2:

$$pH = pK + \log \frac{[HCO_3^-]}{\alpha P_{CO_2}}$$

This is the Henderson–Hasselbalch equation, which relates the three variables. Its value rests in its use to calculate the third variable if any two are known; usually $[HCO_3^-]$ is calculated from measured pH and P_{CO_2}.

More complicated problems

The majority of acid–base problems will be easy to solve once arterial pH and P_{CO_2} have been measured. Why do problems occur and why is acid–base control often presented as such a complicated subject? In essence, problems occur once compensation is complete and it becomes difficult to decide whether the initial perturbation was an abnormality of respiration or of a metabolic component. If, for example, the following measurements were obtained on a patient:

Arterial P_{CO_2} 6.4 kPa (48 mmHg)
pH   7.40
HCO_3^- 29 mmol/l

this situation could be analysed in two ways as a purely acid–base problem (the deviations from normal are sufficiently small that in clinical terms it may be no problem). First, this may be compensated respiratory acidosis; that is, the rise in P_{CO_2} was primary and the small rise in $[HCO_3^-]$ may be attributed to renal compensation. Second, and equally appropriately, it may be that this is a primary metabolic alkalosis and that the rise in P_{CO_2} is secondary. Simple analysis has let us down, and without a more complicated approach we can go no further. Because the problem is a clinical one (albeit the one illustrated is not very pressing), it can probably be solved in clinical terms. This is a step not often allowed for in acid–base analysis. The patient can be examined to discover whether it is likely that a rise in P_{CO_2} occurred (basically a respiratory disorder) or whether a metabolic alkalosis might have occurred (the patient had become hypokalaemic with a consequent metabolic alkalosis).

At this stage it should become clear that problems are relatively infrequent. Acute, simple deviations from normal pH are analysed as in Table 8.3; even when compensation makes the problem more difficult, examining the patient will often solve it. When are more complicated methods of analysing acid–base problems needed? Probably only in two practical situations: to solve the occasional problems which cannot be analysed in the way described, and in an attempt to quantify the acid–base deviation more completely before starting treatment.

Methods of acid-base analysis

The description of the methods of acid–base analysis cannot be detailed, as they are numerous. Any method of analysis, however, is aimed at answering two questions:

1. To determine the extent to which any acid–base abnormality is due to a respiratory or a metabolic disorder.
2. To quantify the acid–base disturbance as a guide to treatment.

There are many individual methods of analysis, but there are two differing approaches which have emerged and which have led to controversy. The first depends on the *in vitro* behaviour of blood. The sample of blood is withdrawn, placed in a tonometer and there the $P\text{CO}_2$ can be changed at will. Measurements can then be made of $[\text{HCO}_3^-]$ or pH at any $P\text{CO}_2$. This allows any respiratory element to be removed *in vitro* by adjustment of the $P\text{CO}_2$ and allows quantification of the metabolic element. The essential measurements made are standard bicarbonate and base excess or deficit. The other approach uses measurements made on arterial blood withdrawn after the whole body equilibrium with CO_2 has been changed *in vivo* (either by breathing CO_2 or by hyperventilation). The proponents of this method emphasize that it is a description of what actually happens in the body. Clearly the *in vitro* method depends on the assumption that the behaviour of blood when equilibrated with CO_2 *in vitro* will give results that do not differ significantly from those which would have occurred *in vivo*. Because the nomograms constructed for using this method were obtained with normal blood, it also depends on the assumption that blood from normals will behave the same way *in vitro* as blood from diseased individuals. The essential measurements are described below and it is worth examining exactly how each measurement is obtained.

Standard bicarbonate

This is the bicarbonate concentration of plasma (in mmol/l) from whole blood which has been equilibrated *in vitro* with a gas mixture which has a $P\text{CO}_2$ of 5.3 kPa (40 mmHg) at 37°C. Essentially, this tells us about the acid–base status of the blood when the respiratory component, which may have existed in the patient, is removed by manipulation of the $P\text{CO}_2$ *in vitro*. In practice, the blood $P\text{CO}_2$ does not have to be equilibrated *in vitro* exactly to a $P\text{CO}_2$ of 5.3 kPa (40 mmHg). The blood is removed and equilibrated at a high $P\text{CO}_2$ and a low $P\text{CO}_2$, the pH is measured at each of these $P\text{CO}_2$s. This will establish the *in vitro* buffer line of the blood being studied and from this can be determined the $[\text{HCO}_3^-]$ at a $P\text{CO}_2$ of 5.3 kPa (40 mmHg)—the standard bicarbonate. If manipulation of the $P\text{CO}_2$ to 5.3 kPa (40 mmHg) produces a normal standard bicarbonate (25 mmol/l), the disturbance must have been solely a respiratory one. If the standard bicarbonate deviates from normal, there is a metabolic component. This can be quantified by measuring base excess (alkalosis) or base deficit (acidosis).

Base excess and base deficit

These are essentially similar derivations. Because an acidosis is usually clinically more important, base deficit will be described. Adjustment of the $P\text{CO}_2$ to 5.3 kPa (40 mmHg), as described above, will have removed the respiratory component. Measurement of the pH at this stage will not reveal the full extent of the acidosis because some of the H^+ will be attached to the buffers of the blood. In order to find out how many H^+ have accumulated they must be released from these buffers. This can be done by titrating the pH of the blood back to 7.40. In the case of an acidosis this is done with NaOH and the base deficit expressed in mmol/l. This depends on the buffer from that sample of blood not differing from the buffer of normal blood and the *in vitro* buffer line being the same as in the *in vivo* buffer line (neither is a justifiable assumption). In an alkalosis the approach is similar; the titration would be performed with HCl, and the value obtained the base excess. In practice these titrations are not, of course, performed but the values obtained from a nomogram relating pH, P_{CO_2}, $[HCO_3^-]$ and Hb. This approach, best described by Siggaard-Anderson (1963), depends on the *in vitro* behaviour of blood.

In vivo techniques

If the equilibration of CO_2 with the whole body is altered, either by breathing CO_2 or by hyperventilation, then the changes in blood pH and $[HCO_3^-]$ can be measured which actually occur *in vivo*. This removes the assumption that equilibration of blood with CO_2 in a tonometer will give the same result as changing P_{CO_2} in the body. Superficially, this seems an attractive approach. The relationship can be established between variation in P_{CO_2} and subsequent changes in pH or $[HCO_3^-]$. If confidence limits are obtained for this relationship, any deviation from them will indicate that the change occurring must be attributed to more than just a change in P_{CO_2}—that is, there must be a metabolic element. Once we have decided to construct *in vivo* relationships, we must obtain one for acute changes in P_{CO_2} and another for chronic changes. The relationship will be different because a chronic respiratory acidosis will produce a renal response, an increase in the excretion of H^+ with a consequent rise in blood $[HCO_3^-]$. Use of the *in vivo* analysis will mean that a different relationship must be used for acute and chronic disorders.

The main difference between the *in vivo* and the *in vitro* approach is summarized in Fig. 8.1. The central curve represents the change in plasma $[HCO_3^-]$ produced by haemoglobin in buffering CO_2 when the blood remains within the tonometer. The acute *in vivo* curve lies below this; again, $[HCO_3^-]$ is produced when the P_{CO_2} is raised but, as the capillary bed is permeable to HCO_3^-, the increase in plasma $[HCO_3^-]$ must be shared with the total ECF. For this reason, *in vivo* there will appear to be a lesser rise in $[HCO_3^-]$ for a given increase in P_{CO_2} than would be the case *in vitro*. If nomograms obtained from *in vitro* results are used, this will lead to the conclusion when analysing results obtained from patients (*in vivo*) that something other than a change in P_{CO_2} has occurred; that is, a metabolic element. This discrepancy depends on a fundamental difference in the modes of analysis.

The third curve in Fig. 8.1 describes the chronic *in vivo* relationship. The change in $[HCO_3^-]$ for a change in P_{CO_2} now depends on renal function as well as haemoglobin buffering; therefore, for a given change in P_{CO_2} there is a change in $[HCO_3^-]$ which is greater than that obtained acutely *in vivo* or *in vitro*. It has already been described why the acute *in vitro* and *in vivo* lines will differ

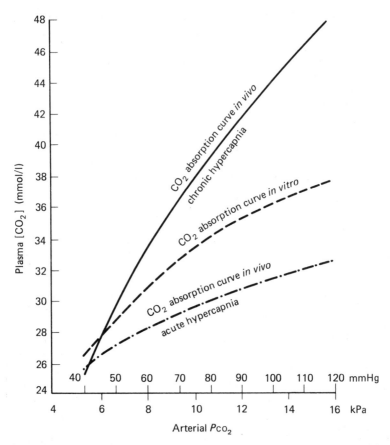

Fig. 8.1 The relationship between plasma [CO_2] and arterial $P\text{co}_2$ *in vitro* and *in vivo*, both acute and chronic. The ordinate represents plasma [CO_2] whereas the text refers to [HCO_3^-]; the relationships will be qualitatively similar because HCO_3^- is the main component of plasma [CO_2]. (Reproduced, with permission, from G. Cumming and S. J. Semple, 1973, *Disorders of the Respiratory System.* Blackwell Scientific, Oxford.)

(this is a fundamental problem). The use of the *in vivo* lines presents another practical problem. It is not always clear clinically whether it is appropriate to use the acute or chronic relationships. This may lead to the diagnosis of a metabolic element which is merely part of the normal compensation. A further deficit of the *in vivo* relationships is that some of the more extreme points (severe hypercapnia and hypocapnia) are obtained on dogs and all the results pertain to *normal* man or animals.

In spite of these theoretical objections, analysis does not present such problems in practice. The reasons for this may be stated quite simply:

1. The accuracy demanded in clinical practice is rarely such that the theoretical problems outlined will invalidate a method *provided* its limitations are realized.

2. The differences between the acute *in vivo* and *in vitro* lines are not large unless the $P\text{CO}_2$ is above 6.7 kPa (50 mmHg).

3. It is possible to correct the *in vitro* nomograms quite simply to give results which make *in vivo* predictions useful if one assumes that the blood volume is diluted by the ECF volume. That is, the effect of haemoglobin is shared between blood and ECF. If *in vitro* nomograms are to be used then a low haematocrit or haemoglobin value should be substituted in the calculations.

It has been pointed out that in spite of the obvious deficiencies in these methods, they are good enough for clinical purposes. This leads to the final section of this chapter which deals with treatment.

Treatment of acid-base disorders

Treatment of an *acidosis* or an *alkalosis* can only be aimed at remedying the basic process before an abnormality of pH develops. No treatment of the acid-base states is required unless there is an alkalaemia or an acidaemia. This section will be mainly about treating a metabolic acidaemia.

Severe metabolic alkalaemia is rare and seldom requires treatment as an acid–base disorder. Most commonly it occurs as a consequence of K^- depletion, and replacement of K^+ (with adequate provision of chloride) suffices to correct the alkalaemia. Rarely, an alkalaemia may require direct action. The general principles are essentially similar to those described for an acidaemia, but ammonium chloride may be used, or, dilute (0.1 mmol/l) hydrochloric acid may be infused into a large central vein.

An acidaemia is a far more common occurrence. If it is a respiratory acidaemia, the primary problem is that of correcting the ventilatory failure (see Chapter 5). The main problem that emerges is treating a metabolic acidaemia. Before treatment is considered, the cause of the metabolic acidaemia will have been diagnosed. Only if the acidaemia is sufficiently severe to be dangerous in its own right should treatment be considered before a definitive diagnosis has been made. The steps to be considered before treatment of an acidaemia is started are:

1. Determine the diagnosis and what steps should be taken to reverse the fundamental disorder.

2. Ascertain whether other abnormalities of electrolyte distribution exist. Often a severe acidaemia will be accompanied by disorders of H_2O, Na^+ and K^+ distribution. These may be more important immediately than the acid-base abnormality. Correction of an acidaemia must always be considered together with requirements for correcting any of these abnormalities.

3. Finally, the treatment of the acidaemia itself.

Correction of the acidaemia is listed last on purpose. Only in a severe acidaemia would such treatment have priority. It is worth discussing in general what degree of acidaemia will require treatment; opinion on this will vary, but two considerations emerge. First, a severe acidaemia will ultimately depress myocardial contractility; after cardiac arrest, correction of the ensuing acidaemia may be necessary before a normal rhythm and output can be established. The acidaemia carries, therefore, dangers in its own right. Second, a severe acidaemia will reflexly stimulate respiration, causing distressing hyperpnoea. The increase in respiration is compensatory, so it is the acidaemia which must be treated and not the hyperventilation. It is difficult to be dogmatic about the levels of arterial pH which require treatment *per se*. Much will depend on the rate at which pH is falling and the general clinical situation. An arterial pH below 7.25 may require treatment, below 7.1 almost certainly will. An arterial pH below 6.95 will, in all probability, be fatal if prolonged at this level.

What is the aim of treatment? Given the limits above for arterial pH, the aim of treatment is to return the arterial pH to a 'safe' value, while attention is directed towards correcting other electrolyte abnormalities and dealing with the basic metabolic defect. If this simple aim is adhered to, relatively simple measures will suffice. It is not necessary, nor is it usually wise, to attempt to correct arterial pH back to normal. Calculations of total base deficit as a basis for such an attempt are usually misleading. These calculations almost invariably overestimate the necessary correction, in diabetic ketoacidosis, possibly by 50 per cent.

What, then, is the practical recommendation for treatment? In the first place, sodium bicarbonate is the wisest choice. Lactate solutions may sometimes be suitable but use of lactate assumes that there is adequate conversion of lactate to pyruvate. This is not true in hepatocellular failure nor if there is a lactic acidosis due to tissue hypoxia. Under these circumstances infusion of lactate will contribute to the lactic acidosis. It is questionable whether there is any case to be made for ever using lactate solutions in view of these potential dangers. The practical course of action is to infuse successive doses of 50–100 mmol of sodium bicarbonate with measurements of arterial pH and $P\text{CO}_2$ before and after until the arterial pH is returned to a 'safe' level. Since the aim of the therapy is limited to this degree of correction, large volumes of sodium bicarbonate are seldom required. If large volumes are required, a further problem arises because the solution of sodium bicarbonate usually available contains 1 mmol of $NaHCO_3$ per millilitre and is therefore hypertonic. If large volumes are infused, there is a danger of sodium overload. Most acidaemias do not require these large amounts of bicarbonate. In a severe lactic acidaemia, however, this is not so and it is wise to use an isotonic solution of sodium bicarbonate as a continuous infusion.

The last important principle is that the correction is better conducted slowly. There are several reasons for this:

1. If the bicarbonate solution is infused rapidly, there may be considerable alkaline transients in blood pH as equilibration occurs. This may lead to severe hypokalaemia as K^+ enters cells, resulting in cardiac arrythmias or to depression of the ionized fraction of Ca^{2+} with consequent tetany or convulsions.

2. Rapid correction may not be increasingly effective if renal function is good, as elevation of plasma $[HCO_3^-]$ above 26–28 mmol will merely exceed the normal renal threshold and increase renal excretion.

3. Rapid correction of blood pH may lead to unexpected effects due to

different rates of equilibration between body compartments. For example, the correction of a metabolic acidaemia will reduce hyperventilation, allowing the arterial P_{CO_2} to rise. Because equilibration of [HCO_3^-] between blood and CSF is slow but that of P_{CO_2} is fast, a situation may arise in which CSF [HCO_3^-] remains low but the P_{CO_2} is rising. A further fall in CSF pH and perhaps in brain tissue pH may occur with consequent impairment of cerebral function. This point may be a theoretical objection to rapid correction of an acidaemia. The dangers of lethal hypokalaemia occurring are more important. Perhaps the best example of this occurs in the treatment of diabetic ketoacidosis. All the major therapeutic steps will reduce plasma [K^-]:

(a) Lowering blood glucose with insulin will increase K^- entry into cells.
(b) Rehydration will lower plasma [K^-] by a dilution effect.
(c) As the acidaemia is corrected by bicarbonate infusion, particularly if the arterial pH is allowed to become alkaline, there will be an increase in the passage of K^- into cells.

If insufficient K^- is infused, dangerous hypokalaemia may ensue. Because the first two steps are essential in the treatment of diabetic ketoacidosis, it is wise to limit the infusion of bicarbonate to the amount necessary to produce a safe arterial pH. An attempt to correct arterial pH to normal will usually result in the infusion of an excess of HCO_3^-. If this is infused rapidly, the dangers are obvious.

The rules, therefore, for treatment of a metabolic acidaemia may be summarized as follows:

1. Only treat a severe acidaemia when the level of arterial pH merits treatment in its own right; otherwise, treat the metabolic defect only.

2. Treat the acidaemia with an infusion of a bicarbonate solution using 50–100 mmol amounts. Repeated measurements of arterial pH must be made to monitor the effects of treatment until the desired effect has been achieved. Thereafter, measurements should be repeated (every 1–2 hours, depending on the clinical setting) to ensure that the treatment of the underlying metabolic disorder is continuing the correction of the acidaemia. If large amounts of sodium bicarbonate are required, there will be a danger of sodium overload.

3. Pay attention:
(a) to the main underlying defect causing the acidaemia;
(b) to the abnormalities of H_2O, Na^+ and K^+ distribution, which may be more important.

4. Design treatment so that correction of arterial pH is achieved over a period of hours. Attempts to correct electrolyte and acid–base disorders in a matter of minutes may lead to severe and life-threatening disequilibria.

9

Pulmonary tuberculosis

In the UK, pulmonary tuberculosis is no longer a common disease, although as a cause of death it once stood in the position of lung cancer today. Nevertheless, a respiratory text without mention of the problems of diagnosing and treating pulmonary tuberculosis is unthinkable. It is worth considering why it remains so important although the incidence of the disease is declining. Partially it is an emotional response; within living memory and before the advent of chemotherapy in the late 1940s and 1950s tuberculosis was a common severe illness in young adults which was often fatal. Many people remember this well and the disease maintains its evil reputation. In spite of effective chemotherapy and a declining incidence, tuberculosis remains a problem. There are still about 1000 deaths each year from tuberculosis in the UK; in about one-third of those who die from this disease the diagnosis was not suspected before death. The way in which we view tuberculosis is influenced by the following points:

1. It was once a widespread and often fatal disease (and not that long ago).
2. In spite of chemotherapy and improved living standards, the disease has not been eradicated.
3. It remains a serious and potentially lethal disease which, if diagnosed early, can be successfully treated.

In the developing countries the situation is vastly different, as tuberculosis remains a serious problem. The annual risk of infection is approximately ten times higher in developing nations than in the more affluent countries of the West. Tuberculosis remains a serious health problem from a world-wide point of view, and it is significant that much of the research on new treatment regimens has originated in the developing countries.

These points show why tuberculosis has been and remains an important topic in chest medicine. There are other reasons why tuberculosis merits a chapter on its own. There is nothing special about the physiology of the disease. Pneumonia caused by the tubercle bacillus will produce the same physiological changes as any other pneumonia. Tuberculosis has, however, certain features which make it unusual:

1. The response to the tubercle bacillus changes after a first infection. This is because cell-mediated hypersensitivity to the organism develops (see later,

the difference between primary and post-primary disease).

2. The tubercle bacillus is extremely slow-growing and hardy. It causes a disease which is chronic and which requires long treatment (months) to eradicate. Herein lie some of the problems. Because it is a chronic disease with an insidious onset, it is possible for infected individuals to continue in the community for a long time and infect others. This would be less likely to happen with an acute explosive infectious disease which prostrated the individual immediately. The long period of chemotherapy necessary for complete treatment poses several problems. Treatment, which used to last for 2 years and now takes 9 months, demands careful supervision and well-motivated patients to achieve compliance. Usually when the patient feels better he stops taking the treatment. The full course of treatment is essential to achieve a complete cure. Lastly, prolonged chemotherapy is expensive; because the disease is commonest among the poor in developing countries, it represents a considerable economic burden.

Epidemiology

Most of the essential points are shown in Fig. 9.1, which gives the annual death rate from tuberculosis in England and Wales from 1915 to 1978. It is salutary to see that a considerable decline in the death rate occurred before the introduction of chemotherapy. This reflects improved health in the community due to better nutrition and housing. Both world wars were accompanied by an increase in the death rate. Finally, there is an obvious

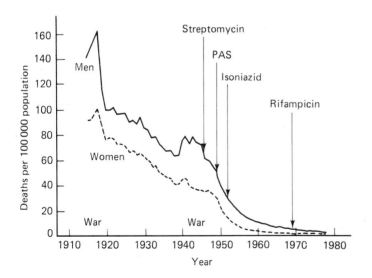

Fig. 9.1 Annual death rate for tuberculosis in England and Wales from 1915 to 1978, showing the rise during each world war but none the less a steady fall, greatly accelerated by classic chemotherapy (streptomycin, PAS and isoniazid). (Reproduced, with permission, from D. C. Flenley, 1981, *Respiratory Medicine*. Baillière Tindall, London.)

impact of chemotherapy but in spite of this there remains a low level of activity of the disease which is now scarcely declining.

The prevalence of tuberculosis can be estimated from the presence of a positive tuberculin test (see below) in the population. Once infected, an individual will have a positive test (even if he has never been clinically ill from tuberculosis). In 1940 approximately 60 per cent of the population of developed countries had been infected; this had fallen to about 25 per cent by 1975. In the UK, approximately 3 per cent of 13-year-old children are tuberculin-positive, whereas in India a positive reaction occurs in 75 per cent of children.

Predisposing factors

Housing conditions
Contagion occurs by inhalation of droplets containing the tubercle bacillus coughed up by an infected individual. Poor housing results in overcrowding which facilitates this process. An infected individual will usually only infect those who are close regular contacts. When tuberculosis is diagnosed, contact tracing should be limited to such individuals; searching more widely among chance contacts is unproductive. The way in which tuberculosis can spread in a closed environment is illustrated by an accident in a submarine. At the time of embarkation on a cruise an infected individual went undiagnosed. Out of the crew of 308, 139 developed a positive tuberculin test (indicating they had been infected). Seven cases of active tuberculosis developed and of these 6 were sailors who slept close to each other and worked as a team. Tuberculosis will always spread when there is overcrowding; the urban slums of developing countries and emergency camps housing refugees form ideal environments for the spread of tuberculosis.

Other concurrent diseases
The risk of tuberculosis is increased in patients already suffering from diabetes, malnutrition, alcoholism and drug dependence. In the UK, tuberculosis is particularly to be suspected in alcoholics and in down-and-outs. Immunosuppression may lead to the development of the disease, whether it is brought about by another disease (leukaemia or Hodgkin's) or by drugs (immunosuppressive treatment after a transplant).

Age
Tuberculosis is commoner in the young and in the very old.

Race
The pattern of tuberculosis varies in different racial groups. Immigrants who have come from areas of high prevalence may be especially at risk.

Reactivation
People who have been infected and appear to have healed, quiescent tuberculous lesions but who have had no, or inadequate, chemotherapy,

represent a residual 'sump' of potential disease. Sometimes these lesions break down and reactivate. The causes of reactivation are related to the predisposing factors listed above—that is, the development of another disease which may debilitate the patient or change his immune state, change in socioeconomic position or the development of alcoholism. One of the ways in which this residual core of potential tuberculosis might be eradicated is by chemo-prophylaxis in individuals known to have been infected (from the chest x-ray) but who have never been adequately treated.

Microbiology and pathology

Tuberculosis is caused by infection with *Mycobacterium tuberculosis*. Infection is generally spread by inhalation of droplets containing this organism coughed by a patient with active disease. The nature of this infection and the identification of this organism was established by Robert Koch in 1882.

There are other forms of mycobacteria which can be infective in man. *Mycobacterium bovis* from cattle is carried in milk from infected cows and presents as intestinal tuberculosis. This is now virtually unknown in developed countries and is becoming increasingly rare in developing countries. There are other atypical mycobacteria which are usually saprophytes but which can occasionally cause disease in man.

The mycobacteria are hardy organisms in the body. Many individuals who have been infected by tuberculosis which has healed without treatment may still have viable organisms in the healed lesion which can, at a later date, reactivate. The aim of chemotherapy is to eradicate all organisms, and to do this the treatment must be prolonged. Conversely, *in vitro*, the organism demands special conditions to grow, and cultures take some 3–6 weeks to develop. This means that after initial culture, and the subculture necessary to obtain *in vitro* sensitivity to drugs, sensitivity will only be available after 10–12 weeks. Because of one of their staining properties, tubercle bacilli are often called acid-fast bacilli (AFBs).

The inhaled droplet containing *M. tuberculosis* is deposited in lung tissue, and in a previously uninfected individual there is an immediate reaction. There is an exudate into the alveolar tissue consisting initially of polymorphs followed by alveolar macrophages and blood monocytes which phagocytose the free bacilli and any polymorphs which contain them. This process produces the epithelioid cells which lie around the inflammatory lesion. This forms the basic lesion of tuberculosis, the tubercle. In this case it is a primary tubercle due to a first infection. At the next stage the tubercle becomes surrounded by lymphocytes. In the 3–8 weeks after the primary infection, one of the key events in the sequence of a tuberculous infection occurs: a cell-mediated hypersensitivity to the proteins of *M. tuberculosis* develops. This alters the response to the bacillus because T-lymphocytes are now sensitized to release lymphokines which will activate macrophages. Once this change has occurred, the nature of the tuberculous lesion changes. It now becomes localized and necrotic in its centre; this is called caseation. Because the centre of the lesion breaks down in this way it often develops into a cavity (in the lung the caseous material containing the bacilli is coughed up). If healing occurs it does so by intense fibrosis, and eventually a healed tuberculous lesion may calcify. Caseation, cavitation, fibrosis and calcification are the hallmarks of tuberculous lesions in the lung.

When cell-mediated hypersensitivity develops, this can be tested for by a positive reaction to an intradermal injection of a protein derived from tubercle bacilli. This is the tuberculin test (see below). Before the development of cell-mediated hypersensitivity, the tubercle bacillus may, in a susceptible individual, spread, causing a disseminated disease (i.e. it behaves like the streptococcus). When hypersensitivity has developed, the response is different; it now produces a localized cavitating lesion (i.e. it behaves like the staphylococcus). Because of this it is essential to distinguish primary tuberculosis in an individual who is not hypersensitive from post-primary tuberculosis in an individual who has developed hypersensitivity. The role of the tuberculin test is central in making this distinction clinically.

The tuberculin test

This is a test to demonstrate the presence or the absence of a reaction to protein derived from the tubercle bacillus. If positive, it indicates that the individual has developed lymphocyte-mediated hypersensitivity to the protein. It can be used diagnostically in an individual and for screening populations.

Two protein derivatives are in common use: a purified protein derivative (PPD), and Koch's old tuberculin. These are used in three forms of tuberculin test, described below.

Mantoux test

In the Mantoux test 0.1 ml of a 1 : 10 000 solution is injected intradermally; this gives a dose of 1 international unit whether PPD or old tuberculin is used. The tuberculin derivative is injected intradermally, usually on the flexor aspect of the arm, together with a control injection. The result is read at 48–72 hours, and is positive if an area of induration of at least 10 mm develops. This test has the advantage that the amount of tuberculin injected can be varied, so that a graded response can be obtained. It is generally used as a diagnostic test in determining whether an individual has had tuberculosis or not.

Heaf test

This test uses a multiple puncture gun; six points are released into the skin when it is fired. Before firing (and after sterilization of the gun), the skin is swabbed with a solution of PPD. When the gun is fired, the needles and PPD penetrate the skin. The result is read after 3–5 days, and a positive reaction occurs if the six separate papules coalesce to form a ring. This method is suitable for carrying out the large numbers of tests necessary in contact tracing and epidemiological surveys.

Tine test

Four prongs 2 mm long are prepared already smeared with old tuberculin; the prongs are pressed hard against the skin and the tuberculin is introduced. Appropriate pressure on the skin is essential and the test is still being evaluated. In terms of convenience, it has great advantages over the other two.

Primary tuberculosis

The initial infection with *M. tuberculosis* will occur as described above. If the initial infection is contained with the host having adequate defences, the primary lesion will develop; this consists of the small pneumonic area in the lung parenchyma with spread to the hilar glands causing their enlargement. The combination of the lesion in the lung and the hilar gland enlargement is called the primary complex. This is particularly common in childhood, and the enlarged hilar glands detected on a chest x-ray may be the only guide to the infection. In adults the glandular element is less obvious.

In most cases the primary complex heals. The only consequence of the infection is a lesion which may remain apparent on the chest x-ray; histologically it is a healed fibrosed tubercle and the individual will become,

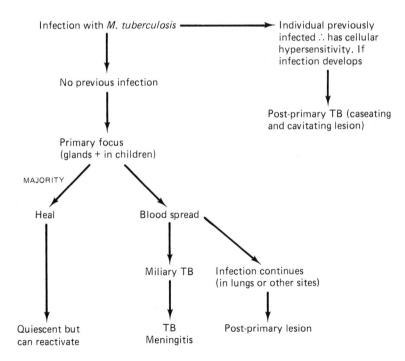

Fig. 9.2 The course of a tuberculous infection.

and remain, tuberculin-positive. In the tubercle the bacilli may be inactive for years; any change in the host (development of another illness or change in immune status) may allow reactivation. The course of primary infection is shown in Fig. 9.2. If healing does not occur, two other sequences may develop as discussed below.

Immediate bloodborne spread

This is a risk particularly in children. Multiple tubercles become disseminated throughout the body, producing miliary tuberculosis. In the lungs this can be seen on the chest x-ray as multiple small opacities distributed throughout the lung fields. The most serious complication of miliary spread is tuberculous meningitis, which is often fatal. Immediate treatment and diagnosis are essential. Examination of the CSF, which may have a high protein content and a predominance of lymphocytes, is crucial. The tubercle bacilli are scanty and found only after careful examination. The consequences of failing to make the diagnosis of tuberculous meningitis are so grave that it is often necessary to initiate treatment on clinical suspicion.

When a tuberculous lesion spreads in this way it usually produces a severe febrile illness, and the patient—usually a child—is extremely ill. Immediate diagnosis and treatment are obviously necessary. Sometimes in the elderly even miliary tuberculosis may produce a less obvious chronic illness.

In contrast with the severe illness of miliary tuberculosis in a child, a primary infection may be scarcely apparent. This must be so, as many people bear the marks of a healed tuberculous lesion on their chest x-ray but are unaware that they ever had such an illness. The primary infection which usually occurs in childhood may be completely unnoticed or may cause only a transient febrile illness.

Intermediate spread

The other consequence of a primary infection which does not heal is an intermediate one. The lesion which has never healed continues and within 2–12 months produces the clinical picture of post-primary tuberculosis. Post-primary tuberculosis, which is the form of tuberculosis after cell-mediated hypersensitivity develops, is a localized disease characterized by caseation and cavitation. As shown in Fig. 9.2, post-primary tuberculosis may arise in three ways:

1. As a continuation of the primary infection after hypersensitivity has developed.

2. As a reactivation of the primary lesion (this may occur years later).

3. Because of reinfection in the patient who has acquired cell-mediated hypersensitivity (probably this is rare).

Post-primary tuberculosis

The clinical picture is one of insidious onset. The individual may be scarcely aware of the illness. Herein lies the danger because it is at this stage that infection may be spread. The classic features of post-primary pulmonary tuberculosis are:

1. Cough.
2. Haemoptysis (coughing up blood).
3. Feeling generally unwell with loss of weight and appetite.
4. Fever.

The diagnosis of tuberculosis is essentially made by isolating the tubercle bacillus. Direct smears of sputum may reveal the presence of tubercle bacilli (acid-fast bacilli on staining) and culture of the sputum will confirm the presence of *M. tuberculosis*. An x-ray of the chest is essential, the typical lesion being a cavitating lesion at the apex of the lung (Fig. 9.3). Sometimes tuberculosis may present simply as pneumonia with no obvious clues other than the failure to improve on standard antibiotics. When this happens, it is essential to examine the sputum for tubercle bacilli.

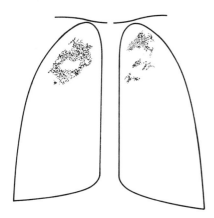

Fig. 9.3   Bilateral apical shadowing with cavitation. This is the typical chest x-ray appearance of post-primary pulmonary tuberculosis.

Lastly, the tuberculin test will help in the diagnosis. In a case of active tuberculosis a strongly positive tuberculin test should be present, provided of course that it is a case of post-primary infection or the infection has been present for more than 6 weeks (the time for the tuberculin sensitivity to develop).

Treatment

With modern treatment regimens, pulmonary tuberculosis is a curable disease. Failure of the disease to respond is attributable to one of the following problems:

1. The infecting organism is not sensitive to the drugs being used.

2. The drugs have not been prescribed in the correct combination or for long enough.

3. The patient is not taking the treatment prescribed.

Chemotherapy of tuberculosis with a single drug was found to lead to relapse and the emergence of resistant strains of tubercle bacilli. The concept was developed of an initial regimen of therapy with three drugs, thus ensuring that the organism would be sensitive to at least two of them. Triple therapy is continued until the results of the sensitivities are known (because the organism is slowly growing this takes about 10 weeks). When the sensitivities are known, the drug which is potentially most toxic can be dropped. Treatment is continued for a long time to ensure that the lesion is sterilized.

The classic regimen for the treatment of pulmonary tuberculosis once consisted of an initial period of treatment (2–3 months) with streptomycin, isoniazid and para-aminosalicylic acid (PAS), followed by treatment with isoniazid and PAS (provided the organism was sensitive) until a 2-year total period of treatment was completed. This regimen was highly effective and the relapse rate after a well supervised course of treatment was low. The disadvantages were the prolonged period of treatment, the toxicity of streptomycin and the rather weak antituberculous action of PAS, which was also extremely unpalatable.

The introduction of rifampicin in 1968 revolutionized the treatment of tuberculosis. It is a powerful bactericidal drug, and has proved so effective that it has allowed short treatment regimens to be developed. Great pressure has come for shorter courses from the developing countries; supervision of a long course of treatment is expensive and a strain on limited medical resources. Trials with various shorter courses in developing countries have led to the following regimen which is now standard:

1. Initially:
   rifampicin 450–600 mg per day depending on body weight
   ethambutol 15 mg/kg body weight per day
   isoniazid 300 mg per day

All three can be given at one time before breakfast on an empty stomach. This initial phase should last for 2 months.

2. Continuation therapy: ethambutol is dropped and therapy continues with rifampicin and isoniazid in the above doses for a further 7 months (9 months' treatment in all).

This regimen has now been carefully proven and is considered standard. It seems likely that shorter courses will be devised which will reduce the total period of treatment to 6 months.

Once treatment has started, it is unlikely that the patient continues to be infectious for very long. This is still a contentious problem but prolonged isolation in hospital seems undesirable nowadays. If social circumstances will allow, once diagnosed the patient is best treated at home. Prolonged periods of enforced rest are unnecessary with modern chemotherapy. Even the most conservative agree that after 1 month of chemotherapy with the triple therapy outlined above the patient is no longer infectious. Tubercle bacilli may still be found in the sputum but they are mostly non-viable and unable to infect another individual. Some people suspect that this becomes true after only 1-2 weeks of treatment. Tuberculosis is no longer, therefore, a disease which takes people away from their home and work for 2 years. At the most, a month of isolation may be necessary (but this need not be so if the patient can stay at home). Home treatment carries the advantage that the family will be screened anyway and does not remove the patient at his most infective to a new environment.

The drugs used in the treatment of tuberculosis—rifampicin, ethambutol and isoniazid—may have serious side effects.

1. Rifampicin. At the beginning of treatment, anorexia, nausea and vomiting may occur. The urine becomes orange-red. Early in treatment there may be a rise in the blood levels of various liver enzymes but these usually return to normal even if the drug is continued. Occasionally, severe hepatitis with jaundice may occur but this is rare (less than 1 per cent of cases receiving rifampicin).

2. Ethambutol. The main side effect is the occurrence of an optic neuritis; this occurs with doses in excess of 15 mg/kg body weight per day. Patients on ethambutol should always be asked to report visual disturbances.

3. Isoniazid. Side effects are rare, a peripheral neuropathy being the most dramatic. This can be prevented by giving pyridoxine with the isoniazid. Sometimes isoniazid can give rise to a drug fever, a drug-induced rash or enlarged lymph glands.

Other antituberculous drugs exist. Their use is beyond the scope of this book but they are mainly of value when the infecting organism is resistant to one (or more) of the main drugs. Drug resistance has not turned out to be the problem which was once feared. Primary drug resistance, when a patient has never had antituberculous chemotherapy, occurs in about 4 per cent of cases in developed countries. In developing countries where therapy may be less adequately controlled this figure rises to about 10 per cent. Secondary drug resistance occurs when the organisms become resistant during the course of treatment. This indicates an inadequate regimen or poor compliance on the patient's part. Although this is rare, it is important because infection transmitted from such a patient leads to cases of primary drug resistance.

Prevention

At the beginning of this chapter it was said that the spread of tuberculosis was aided by overcrowding, poor nutrition and poverty. Perhaps the most important preventive measure is general concern with the welfare of the community. The following specific measures are available and should be used rigorously.

Contact tracing

Tuberculosis is a notifiable disease. Once it has been notified, the chest clinic concerned will take steps to identify and screen the contacts of the known patient. This is aimed at discovering those whom he has infected and/or the source of his infection. The tools of screening are the tuberculin test and the chest x-ray. Conversion of the tuberculin test in a contact is evidence of infection and warrants treatment. If the tuberculin test of a known contact is found to be negative 6 weeks after exposure (i.e. long enough for the hypersensitivity to develop) then protection with BCG is indicated (see below). Contacts with a positive tuberculin test should also have a chest x-ray. Children who are contacts should be examined very carefully in the same way.

Population screening

In the UK mass miniature radiography (MMR) was used. This was effective in terms of pick-up when tuberculosis was more prevalent. The pick-up from this technique now is so low in the UK that it is being discontinued. Screening may still be of value for those in prison, institutions or among alcoholics who are particularly at risk. Similarly, screening immigrants is also useful, particularly those coming from areas where tuberculosis is common.

Bacille Calmette–Guérin (BCG)

The aim of vaccination with BCG (a live attenuated strain) is to produce increased resistance to the disease by inducing cell-mediated immunity. After BCG vaccination the tuberculin test will convert and become positive.

In the UK, BCG vaccination is offered to all tuberculin-negative 13-year-olds. BCG vaccination reduces the risk of developing tuberculosis and provides an 80 per cent protection rate for a period up to 10 years. BCG vaccination is also offered to tuberculin-negative persons who are at risk of meeting infected individuals; that is, nurses, laboratory technicians and doctors. BCG may also be used in tuberculin-negative contacts of known cases, such as the babies of mothers suffering from tuberculosis. In spite of the proven value of BCG in the UK, a recent trial in South India failed to confirm the protection for that population. Further trials may be needed to sort this out.

Tuberculosis has been successfully combated and reduced to a low level in the UK compared with the position some 30–40 years ago. These steps have not proved sufficient to eradicate the disease and a 'sump' of the disease remains. Because of this, cases are not uncommon and it is a diagnosis which can be easily overlooked. The message must be, therefore, one of constant awareness of the disease, remembering that in a high proportion of those dying of tuberculosis, the possibility of this treatable condition was not considered.

10

Carcinoma of the bronchus

It might seem strange to include this chapter in a book dedicated to the physiological principles in medicine but carcinoma of the bronchus refuses to be confined by the boundaries imposed by the titles of the other chapters and is too important to omit from any book on chest disease. In 1976 it killed more than 25 000 men and 5000 women in England, Wales and Scotland, more than 90 000 men and women in the USA and the annual mortality in both sexes continues to rise. This is more than four times the annual death rate from road traffic accidents and accounts for around 1 in 10 of the men who died aged 45 or more. Perhaps more depressing is the fact that most of the patients with carcinoma of the bronchus are dead within 12 months of diagnosis, whatever treatment is offered. A study of the natural history of carcinoma of the bronchus indicates why this sorry state of affairs is likely to remain unaltered until adequate preventive measures are taken or entirely new methods of treatment devised.

Know your adversary: the properties of tumour cells

Tumour cells differ from normal cells in two important ways. They are long-lived and they can invade and destroy normal tissue.

If a mass of cells is to accumulate, the rates of the production or of the decay of the constituent cells must alter. If cells are produced faster than they die, the cells accumulate. If the life of a cell type is prolonged and production remains constant, accumulation occurs. When a cell alters its properties in either way, a 'tumour' results. The following paragraphs explore the problems of cell kinetics, degree of differentiation and the special properties which cause problems in the diagnosis and treatment of carcinoma of the bronchus.

Cell kinetics of carcinoma of the bronchus

In the development of the embryo, pluripotential cells differentiate to form tissues and their rate of division falls to the extent that many of the cells of mature tissues no longer divide. When cells of a mature tissue escape from the mechanisms controlling their division and assume their natural replication unchecked, a mass will form. If no cells die, the rate at which this mass increases in size will be described by an exponential function, for the repeated doubling of the number of cells describes a geometric progression. In clinical terms this is illustrated by following the progress of a tumour which starts as a single cell with a division rate of once every 100 days. After a year there will be 8 cells, after 2 years 256 cells, after 5 years 3.1×10^5 cells, and after 8 years 6.2×10^8 cells. This is converted into tumour weight in Table 10.1. The average tumour load at death is estimated to be 1 kg. If a tumour is spherical,

Table 10.1   The gain in weight of a tumour starting with a single cell weighing 1×10^{-5} g which divides once every 100 days, assuming no cells die

Growth time (years)	Weight (g)
0	1×10^{-5}
1	1.3×10^{-4}
2	1.6×10^{-3}
3	2.0×10^{-2}
4	2.5×10^{-1}
5	3.1
6	39
7	490
7.3	1000 (1 kg)

a 1 kg tumour would have a diameter of 10 cm and would result from 7 years and 4 months of unrestrained division of the single cell. In most patients the carcinoma of the bronchus measures about 3 cm in diameter when the diagnosis is made. This represents 6 years' growth. The tumour is rarely detected until it is 1 cm in diameter after 4½ years' growth.

These figures highlight the problem faced by the clinician when treating carcinoma of the bronchus. The example above had a division or doubling time of 100 days. The three most common histological types of carcinoma of the bronchus—squamous carcinoma, small cell carcinoma and adeno-carcinoma—have doubling times of 30–160 days. The 30-day tumour (small cell carcinoma) reaches 1 cm in diameter in 2 years 6 months and the 160-day tumour (adenocarcinoma) 13 years. This represents the interval of tumour growth during which there is little chance that it will be detectable by normal means. If smoking were abolished tomorrow the incidence of newly diagnosed small cell carcinoma (30 days) would not fall for nearly 3 years, and squamous carcinoma (90 days) for over 7 years. Surveys of doctors who gave up smoking have been carried out by Professor Doll and his colleagues over the past 30 years and have shown that predictions based on these assumptions are close to the truth. By the time the patient presents, he is in the late phase of the natural history of the tumour and it is not surprising that therapeutic intervention is so rarely curative.

The cells of the basal layers of the skin and the gut and those producing the red and white blood cells in the bone marrow divide more rapidly than any of the types of the carcinoma of the bronchus. It is not the rapidity with which tumour cells multiply which causes their accumulation; it is the fact that they do not stop dividing and are very long-lived.

As the pluripotential embryonic cell differentiates, its rate of division slows and life span becomes finite. Tumours show a similar gradation of properties. The less well differentiated the tumour the more rapidly the cells divide, shown by the number of mitoses in histological preparations, and the greater the proportion of the cells of the tumour which will continue to divide. The less differentiated the tumour, the shorter the doubling time.

Modes of spread: the properties of invasion and migration

An even more unpleasant property acquired by poorly differentiated tumour cells is the ability to invade tissues and to break from the site of origin, float away in tissue fluids and continue to divide wherever they lodge. The capacity to invade and spread by distant seeding, metastasizing, is more marked in the poorly differentiated tumour.

Table 10.2 Spread of carcinoma of the bronchus

Structure involved	Problem produced
Expansion at the primary site: local	
Peripheral:	
Pleura	Pleural effusion
Chest wall	Bone pain
	Pain referred down infiltrated nerves: intercostal, brachial plexus
Central:	
Trachea	Stridor and breathlessness
Oesophagus	Dysphagia
Pericardium	Effusion
Spread by circulating fluids: metastatic	
Lymphatic	Regional nodes in hilum then to mediastinal and supraclavicular nodes
	Lymphangitis carcinomatosa (growth down lung lymphatic channels)
Blood stream	Pulmonary metastases
	Systemic metastases (preferred sites: brain, bone marrow, liver)

Table 10.2 lists the possible modes of spread of carcinoma of the bronchus. Spread occurs at the primary site (where the tumour arose) by expansion of the mass of cells or by invasion of local structures. If the tumour occurs in the periphery of the lung, it can invade the chest wall or the pleura. The most dramatic example of chest wall invasion is a tumour at the apex of the lung which invades the brachial plexus, leading to severe pain in the arm and weakness of the hand. This is called the superior sulcus syndrome. Pleural spread causes an accumulation of fluid in the pleural space, and tumour cells are shed into the fluid to drift to a new site, seeding the pleura at a distance. Spread is discontinuous so sampling of fluid or pleura may not yield

diagnostically valuable material. Tumours close to the mediastinum can invade any of the important structures in the immediate vicinity, leading to constriction of the hollow tubes (trachea, bronchi, oesophagus), block of the nerves (recurrent laryngeal nerve, hoarse voice; phrenic nerve, paralysed diaphragm) or invasion of blood vessels. If the veins draining into the right atrium are invaded, metastases or tumour masses developing as a result of discontinuous spread occur in the lung. If the clumps of tumour cells are released into the systemic circulation by transmission through the lungs or by invasion of the pulmonary veins, metastases occur in the capillary beds of the systemic circulation. The organs most often involved by metastases from primary carcinoma of the bronchus are brain, liver, bone marrow and suprarenal glands. The reasons for this distribution are not entirely clear. The frequent involvement of the brain could be explained by the fact that it takes 30 per cent of the resting cardiac output, but this cannot account for the frequency with which the adrenal is involved and is obviously not the only factor since metastases are less frequent in the kidneys which also have a large blood flow.

The cell type and degree of differentiation of the tumour will determine how rapidly it spreads. If the tumour is well differentiated, it grows slowly and has a long silent interval before being clinically detectable at the primary site (see above) but it invades slowly and metastasizes late. This explains why the slow-growing squamous carcinoma has the highest 'cure' or 10-year survival after surgical resection of the primary tumour. It also explains why the prognosis (outlook for survival) for small cell or anaplastic large cell carcinomas, both of which divide rapidly and are poorly differentiated, is unaffected by surgery or local radiotherapy to the primary tumour. In these cases it is the metastases in the brain, bone and liver which determine survival.

Knowledge of the cell type and degree of differentiation of a carcinoma of the bronchus would be of academic interest only if no therapy were available. However, the modern clinician can call on many powerful and uncomfortable means of treatment. Thoracotomy and removal of the primary tumour is an inappropriate procedure for a patient who will die of distant metastases. Failure to remove a resectable well differentiated squamous carcinoma of the bronchus or to give radical radiotherapy may miss the chance of 'cure'. Only when the natural history of the different tumours is understood will rational therapeutic decisions be made.

Special properties of some tumours

A few tumours cause changes in the patient, which can be recognized long before the primary tumour mass has reached a size detectable by normal diagnostic means. Some of these are listed in Table 10.3. It is easiest to explain those associated with recognizable hormones. During embryonic development a group of cells originating in the neural crest migrates to the wall of the gut and its related structures. They are histologically recognizable by silver staining (argentaffin cells) or electron microscopy and are the origin of many hormones. Their function in the lung has been little studied. A tumour of these cells is a small cell or oat cell carcinoma, and most of the endocrine

Table 10.3   Non-metastatic manifestations of carcinoma of the bronchus

Manifestation	Effect
Recognizable endocrine syndromes	
Antidiuretic hormone	Hyponatraemia
Adrenocorticotrophic hormone	Cushing's syndrome Hypokalaemia
Parathyroid hormone	Hypercalcaemia
Thyroid-stimulating hormone	Hyperthyroidism
Serotonin	Carcinoid syndrome
Other manifestations	
General	Anorexia and weight loss Hypoglycaemia
Neurological	Dementia Cerebellar ataxia Spinal cord degeneration Peripheral neuropathy Mononeuritis multiplex
Muscular	Polymyositis Myasthenic syndrome
Vascular	Thrombophlebitis Non-infective endocarditis
Haematological	Thrombocytopenia, thrombocytosis Haemolytic anaemia
Oddities	Clubbing of fingers Hypertrophic pulmonary osteoarthropathy

syndromes are associated with this cell type. Tumour cells may secrete poly-peptides which have no hormonal activity, either because they are improperly constructed or because they have no recognizable link with the endocrine system. These products may be recognized and used to detect tumours which are difficult to find by normal means. Examples of this are chorioncarcinoma of the uterus which secretes human chorionic gonadotrophin (HCG) and some colonic carcinomas which secrete carcinoembryonic antigen (CEA). Unfortunately, carcinoma of the bronchus produces no circulating product as yet recognized which will allow early and reliable detection. It should be noted that some syndromes caused by carcinoma of the bronchus are produced by circulating hormones which are immunologically distinct from normal hormone. This is true of some cases of Cushing's syndrome where adrenocorticotrophic hormone (ACTH) immunologically distinguishable from normal ACTH is circulating, and many cases of hypercalcaemia where no circulating parathyroid hormone can be detected yet no other cause for the hypercalcaemia can be found. It is probable that many of the other syndromes or clinical effects listed in Table 10.3 are produced by circulating tumour products which are unrecognized.

Detection of tumours

Screening of asymptomatic individuals

There is no evidence that screening of asymptomatic individuals affects the prognosis of patients with carcinoma of the bronchus by detecting the disease early in its course. An attempt was made to use the mass radiography service to detect early cases but the chest x-ray will only detect a carcinoma of the bronchus in the late stages of the disease and this has been a failure. There is no 'tumour marker' or substance present in high concentration in the circulating blood specific for lung tumours and no recognizable change in the pattern of normal blood constitutents. Study of the sputum of healthy individuals, looking for shed tumour cells, has been equally unrewarding.

Diagnosis

History
Suspicion that the patient has a carcinoma of the bronchus should be aroused by several symptoms. The most important are coughing blood (haemoptysis) and weight loss in a patient who smokes cigarettes. Repeated attacks of pneumonia—cough and sputum, fever and pleuritic pain (pain over the affected lung, worse on inspiration or coughing)—in the same segment or lobe of lung or a pneumonia which is slow to resolve require further investigation. All tumours have a long asymptomatic period and may be detected by chance during this interval (see above).

Examination
Unless the primary tumour is positioned to produce partial or complete occlusion of one of the main bronchi, it is unusual to find abnormal signs in the chest. If a large bronchus is partly occluded, a musical wheeze may be heard over that lobe of the lung; if the bronchus is totally occluded, consolidation and collapse of the lobe follow and the wheeze disappears. Pleural effusions, paralysis of the diaphragm or recurrent laryngeal nerve palsy produce characteristic signs. Other signs strongly suggestive of a carcinoma of the bronchus are clubbing of the finger nails, palpable metastases in lymph nodes or the signs associated with cerebral or liver metastases. However, none of these is present solely in carcinoma of the bronchus and can only lead the clinician to make the diagnosis by further investigations.

Investigations
Further investigation of the patient is necessary:

1. To confirm the diagnosis.
2. To establish the histological variety of lung tumour.
3. To assess whether the tumour has spread from the primary site.

The scheme of investigation suggested in Fig. 10.1 is a progression from simple and safe procedures to the major step of submitting the patient to an

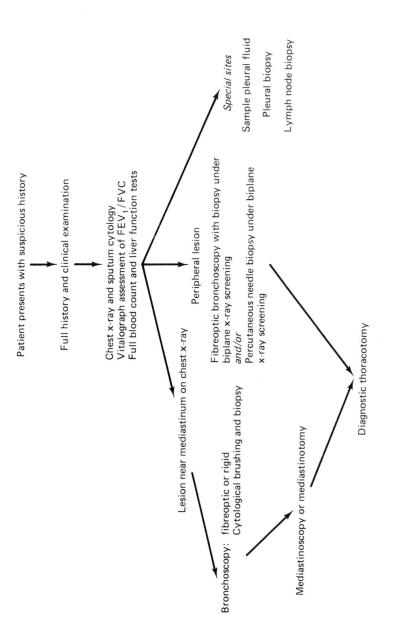

Fig. 10.1 Investigation of a patient with carcinoma of the bronchus. As soon as the diagnosis is confirmed and the extent of spread determined, further investigation is unnecessary.

exploratory thoracotomy. When the three aims above are satisfied, treatment can be planned and further investigation becomes unnecessary. The diagnosis may be obvious when the patient presents with a widespread tumour, has a typical chest x-ray and diagnostic sputum cytology but it may be necessary to proceed to diagnostic thoracotomy before investigation is complete because it is imperative to have histological proof of the diagnosis.

Chest x-ray   The first investigation which should be performed on all patients in whom carcinoma of the bronchus is suspected is a chest x-ray. This may show a shadow which could be a primary tumour in the lung or may be one of the many other causes of shadowing in the lung field (Fig. 10.2b). A mass which has strands of tissue extending into the surrounding lung, contains no calcification and is associated with enlargement of the regional lymph nodes is highly suspicious. If the tumour outgrows its blood supply, the middle of the tumour mass will die. When this happens in the lung, the necrotic central tissue liquefies and is expectorated leaving a cavity which may contain a fluid level (Fig. 10.2c). When this appearance is seen the sputum is copious, often foul-smelling and usually contains neoplastic cells (see below). Other

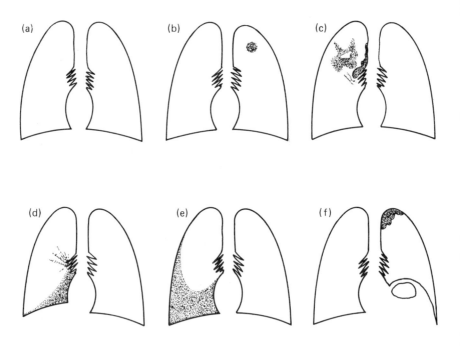

Fig. 10.2 Chest x-ray appearances of a primary carcinoma of the bronchus. (a) Normal. (b) Solitary shadow on otherwise normal chest x-ray. (c) Peripheral tumour with cavity and fluid level, and hilar and paratracheal node involvement. (d) Tumour of large bronchus with lobar collapse (right lower lobe and middle lobe collapse). (e) Pleural effusion. (f) Left phrenic nerve involvement from apical tumour. See text for further details.

complications which produce characteristic chest x-ray appearances are lobar collapse (Fig. 10.2d), pleural effusion (Fig. 10.2e) and diaphragmatic paralysis due to phrenic nerve involvement by invasion of mediastinal tissue by primary or secondary tumour (Fig. 10.2f). Figure 10.2a is included because a normal chest radiograph does *not* exclude a bronchial carcinoma, and it should be remembered that even the chest x-ray which appears 'classic' can be caused by other tumours or by non-malignant diseases. Cytological or histological proof is necessary to confirm the diagnosis and to determine rational treatment.

Cytology Characteristic neoplastic cells may be found in the sputum. This is a useful examination if care is taken in the provision and collection of specimens (sputum from the trachea or bronchi, not saliva) and there is an expert cytologist to interpret the slides. Cytology of the sputum has the advantage that it is not invasive and can be repeated easily, but poor specimen collection is a frequent cause of false-negative results and makes the cytologist's task impossible. Cytology can also be performed on pleural fluid but malignant pleural effusions are frequently blood-stained, making it difficult to pick out the few shed malignant cells.

Bronchoscopy Rigid bronchoscopy is a procedure which should be performed under general anaesthetic, and can be used to assess tumours in the trachea or large bronchi. Since the fibreoptic bronchoscope became available it has become possible to visualize and to biopsy a lesion in any segmental bronchus of any lobe of the lung as well as those in the central airways. It is also possible to biopsy lesions in the periphery of the lung beyond the vision of the bronchoscopist, using x-ray screening to ensure that the lesion is biopsied. This can be done under local anaesthetic on patients attending hospital as outpatients. Samples of the tumour can be taken using a stiff nylon brush (yields a cytology specimen) or biopsy forceps (yields histological samples). It is common practice to take samples of both sorts from every lesion because this increases the diagnostic yield. Such procedures can be carried out under local or general anaesthetic, are safe (mortality: 1 in 8000) and have a high chance of confirming the diagnosis by visualizing the tumour and providing histological proof (more than 80 per cent accurate in patients eventually proved to have carcinoma of the bronchus). Fibreoptic bronchoscopy is the investigation of choice in patients suspected of having a lung tumour.

Further specialized investigations If bronchoscopy fails to prove the diagnosis and to determine the extent of the tumour, further investigations may be required (Table 10.4). Because some of these involve operative procedures, they are undertaken only when simpler measures have failed to prove the diagnosis or determine management. For example, a patient who has a small localized well differentiated squamous carcinoma with no clinical evidence of metastases needs to have a careful neurological examination, liver function tests and a bone scan as the most sensitive ways of looking for occult metastases. Whether such patients need to have a CT scan of the thorax (computerized axial tomography, a special radiological investigation) and a

Table 10.4   Assessment of extent of spread of carcinoma of the bronchus

Problem	Investigation
Liver metastases	Liver function tests, isotopic liver scan, liver ultrasound, liver biopsy
Bone metastases	Blood alkaline phosphatase Isotopic bone scan
Cerebral metastases	Isotopic brain scan or CT scan of the head
Pleural spread	Pleural tap Pleural biopsy
Involvement of palpable lymph glands	Lymph node biopsy
Mediastinal spread	Tomography of mediastinum or CT scan of the thorax ↓ Mediastinoscopy or mediastinotomy

mediastinoscopy prior to having their lung removed (pneumonectomy) is debated but both could be justified. Conversely, a patient presenting with mediastinal and supraclavicular nodes and clinical cerebral metastases needs the minimum of investigation prior to palliative treatment, as a cure cannot be achieved. The principles discussed early in this chapter emphasize that knowledge of the histological type of the tumour is necessary because this determines the probability of distant metastases being present at the time of diagnosis and hence the possibility of 'cure' by local treatment. Systemic chemotherapy or simple palliation are indicated for disseminated disease (see below).

Treatment

Once the diagnosis is confirmed, the three major types of treatment currently available for the patient with carcinoma of the bronchus are:

1. Surgery.
2. Radiotherapy.
3. Intravenous or oral chemotherapy.

Each has its place in the management of the treatable patient.

Surgery

Surgery which removes all of the tumour can be curative and is the ideal treatment. From the preceding pages it must be apparent that the vast majority of patients with carcinoma of the bronchus have tumour present in the lymph nodes of the mediastinum or in other organs outside the lung, rendering cure by removal of one lung impossible. However, there is one group of patients in whom every effort should be made to establish whether the disease has remained confined to one lung. In patients with well differentiated squamous carcinoma of the bronchus the tumour grows slowly and metastasizes late in its course. Those patients who have operable tumour—that is, a tumour which can be completely removed leaving enough bronchus to establish satisfactory closure—and who could withstand the loss of one lobe of the lung or one lung, should have surgery. The 5-year survival for this small group is raised from 2 out of 10 to 4 out of 10 by appropriate lung resection. There is no evidence that surgery for large cell anaplastic carcinoma or small cell carcinoma alters the prognosis because even technically operable tumours are accompanied by distant metastases in the vast majority of cases. Thoracotomy has its own mortality (between 5 and 10 per cent) and morbidity (pain, postoperative breathlessness and a month in hospital or convalescent), and should not be offered to those it has no chance of curing.

The place of surgery in the diagnosis of suspected tumours has been discussed. Whether removal of the primary tumour mass prior to systemic chemotherapy will turn out to prolong survival has yet to be determined.

Radiotherapy

Ionizing radiation in appropriate dosage kills dividing cells. This property is used in the sterilization of food products and in the treatment of disease. If the correct dose is delivered to a tumour, the cells in the path of the radiation beam will be destroyed by disruption of the DNA in the nucleus. However, this is not an effect confined to tumour cells and any dividing cell is susceptible to x-rays. When the radiation beam is used to treat lung tumours, it must pass through skin and will impinge upon bones rich in haemopoietic tissue. The toxic effects on skin and bone marrow limit the dose of irradiation that can be given to the carcinoma of the bronchus. The second property which limits dosage is the inevitable destruction of small blood vessels—radiation vasculitis. This causes the death of tissues which receive large doses of ionizing radiation, and is a major cause of the damage to the skin and the normal lung tissue inevitable in treating lung tumours with radiotherapy. Despite these problems, radiotherapy produces regression of tumours (assessed by repeated chest x-rays) and may improve long-term survival in squamous carcinoma of the bronchus.

Radiotherapy can be used to attempt cure (radical radiotherapy) in those patients who have squamous carcinoma and are inoperable because of the position of the tumour or for other reasons such as poor pulmonary reserve (exercise breathlessness and an FEV_1 of less than 1.5 litres).

The side effects of radiotherapy limit the beam size or field which can be used and therefore confine the area which can be treated. This means that disseminated carcinoma cannot be eradicated using ionizing radiation. Progress in the use of ionizing radiation to cure carcinoma will depend upon making tumour cells more sensitive to its effects. Attempts to do this using hyperbaric oxygen to improve tumour oxygenation have not been successful but there is hope that chemically sensitizing the tumour by treatment of the patient with a drug taken up by the tumour cell (e.g. misonidazole) will be more successful.

Radiotherapy can be used to treat particular areas of tumour cells which cause symptoms by growing in vulnerable sites even when there is no chance of cure (palliative radiotherapy). The treatment of cerebral metastases or of deposits of tumour causing pain by growing in bone is very successful. It can also reduce haemoptysis and relieve superior vena cava obstruction. None of these will prolong survival but the treatment is invaluable as it alleviates pain and reduces distress.

Chemotherapy

Many chemicals have been shown to kill dividing cells. The problem faced by the chemotherapist is the same as that faced by the radiotherapist. Small doses do no harm to the patient but do not affect the tumour, and large doses cure the tumour but kill the patient. To overcome this problem the idea of multiple drug therapy given at intervals was developed. Drugs acting on cells in different ways are given in·doses which harm the tumour and normal dividing cells alike. The combination of the drugs is chosen from those known to have activity against the particular tumour to be treated in order to minimize the effect on normal tissues. The normal tissues and the tumour both recover in the interval between the treatments but the normal tissues recover faster. In this way repeated doses harmful to the tumour but relatively harmless to bone marrow, skin and gut epithelium may be given.

The advantage of chemotherapy is that it is distributed throughout the body by the blood stream. It is the method of choice for treating disseminated disease. Delivery is dependent on the blood supply, so large poorly perfused tumour masses are less well treated than micrometastases. The most serious disadvantages are nausea and vomiting following the injections (variable but sometimes so severe that the treatment has to be stopped) and bone marrow suppression. The latter renders the patient susceptible to infection and is a very serious problem. A comprehensive list of chemotherapeutic agents is outside the scope of this book but those commonly used in carcinoma of the bronchus are listed in Table 10.5. These are most useful in the treatment of small cell carcinoma of the bronchus where chemotherapy has improved median survival (50 per cent of patients still alive) from about 3

Table 10.5   Principal chemotherapeutic agents used in small cell carcinoma of the bronchus

Class (and drug)	Principal toxicity
Antimetabolites (e.g. methotrexate)	Bone marrow suppression Oral ulceration
Vinca alkaloids (e.g. vincristine)	Peripheral neuropathy
Alkylating agents (e.g. cyclophosphamide)	Bone marrow suppression Chemical cystitis
Antitumour antibiotics (e.g. doxorubicin, Adriamycin)	Bone marrow suppression Cardiotoxicity
Podophyllotoxin (e.g. etoposide)	Bone marrow suppression

months to 10 months and a few patients with a small tumour load at the time of diagnosis may survive more than 2 years.

It is obvious from this discussion that none of these treatments is likely to be universally applicable to all cases of carcinoma of the bronchus. Combinations of surgery and chemotherapy or chemotherapy and radiotherapy are required for many tumours. The combined experience of the chest physician, the thoracic surgeon, the radiotherapist and the oncologist gives the patient the best chance of rational treatment and survival.

These are the treatments in current use, and the dismal fact that despite these often heroic efforts fewer than 5 of 100 patients presenting with carcinoma of the bronchus will be alive 5 years after diagnosis shows their inadequacy. Are there any new treatments in prospect? We have learned from studies of carcinoma of the breast and by applying the knowledge gained in the rapidly advancing field of immunology that many tumours are destroyed or contained by the body's immune system. This raises two possibilities for future treatment. The first is to sensitize the body's lymphocytes to the tumour and to induce them to treat the tumour as 'foreign'. This would lead to destruction of the tumour and cure. The second is to attach drugs to γ-globulin molecules targeted onto the tumour. This would enable high doses of drug to be concentrated in the tumour cells, limiting general toxicity. Both hold exciting prospects but are not currently available. The best hope of counteracting the epidemic of lung cancer in the foreseeable future lies in prevention.

Prevention

The principle of prevention implies that the cause of the problem is known. Certain causative factors of carcinoma of the bronchus are known. Three of the histological varieties of lung cancer—squamous (55 per cent of all lung primary carcinoma), small cell (20 per cent) and large cell anaplastic (10 per cent)—are all strongly linked to cigarette consumption. These may occur in non-smokers but a man or woman smoking 25 or more cigarettes per day has a 30 times higher chance of dying of carcinoma of the bronchus and ex-smokers who have stopped for 5 years or more still have three times the chance of the lifelong non-smoker. The prevention of smoking, particularly of cigarettes, is the single most important way of reducing carcinoma of the bronchus. There is a popular belief that it is impossible to stop patients smoking, but there is evidence that this is untrue. In Finland the government has banned cigarette advertising and has undertaken to increase the tax on tobacco annually. This has coincided with a 9 per cent fall in male adult smoking rates in 5 years. This demonstrates that determined campaigns work. The British government is not yet willing to support such a programme. Individuals or groups can be convinced in other ways. The smoking among male British doctors has fallen from an average of 9 cigarettes per doctor per day in 1951 to 3 in 1971. The proportion of non-smokers in this group has risen from 17 per cent in 1951 to 75 per cent in 1971. During this period of 20 years the cigarette consumption of the nation rose. This motivated group has succeeded in cutting its tobacco consumption and sets an example for the patients attending their clinics who claim that they cannot give up smoking. This group has seen a steady fall in the incidence of carcinoma of the bronchus during the study period. It suggests that more attention to preventing people from smoking would have a greater effect on the mortality from lung cancer than any other measure currently available.

Besides smoking there are other factors which can be shown to cause carcinoma of the bronchus. They have a smaller effect in numerical terms but should not be ignored. They are atmospheric pollution, working with certain materials such as asbestos and haematite and inhaling the dust, and possibly scarring diseases of the lung. Public health measures such as wearing masks while processing dangerous materials and ventilating factories are the obvious ways to attack this problem.

Non-smoking-related carcinoma of the bronchus, adenocarcinoma (10 per cent of all bronchial carcinoma) and alveolar cell carcinoma (1 per cent) will be more difficult to prevent because the aetiology is unknown.

The future

Prevention of the tumours and new selective forms of treatment provide the best chance of reducing the rising mortality from carcinoma of the bronchus. We must look to immunology as the most likely source of new treatment, but prevention could be tackled now by abolishing smoking. Many forms of carcinoma of the bronchus are preventable, and urgent action is needed to convince government and the public that stopping smoking would slash the incidence of this unpleasant disease.

Further reading

It is assumed that the reader is familiar with the companion volume, John Widdicombe and Andrew Davies (1983) *Respiratory Physiology*. Edward Arnold, London.

General

Bates, D. V., Macklem, P. T. and Christie, R. V. (1971) *Respiratory Function in Disease*, 2nd edn. W. B. Saunders, Philadelphia.
   A classic text relating disease processes to function. An excellent first section on lung function tests.
Cotes, J. E. (1975) *Lung Function: Assessment and Application in Medicine*, 3rd edn. Blackwell Scientific, Oxford.
   A classic of applied respiratory physiology. Detailed descriptions of all lung function tests, their uses and shortcomings.
Crofton, J. and Douglas, A. (1981) *Respiratory Diseases*, 3rd edn. Blackwell Scientific, Oxford.
   The standard UK textbook of respiratory diseases and their treatment.
Dunnill, M. S. (1982) *Pulmonary Pathology*. Churchill Livingstone, Edinburgh.
   New textbook of pathology, readable.
Flenley, D. C. (1981) *Respiratory Medicine*. Ballière Tindall, London.
   A first-class up-to-date paperback on respiratory diseases.
Spencer, H. (1977) *Pathology of the Lung*, 3rd edn. Pergamon, Oxford.
   Reference work on lung pathology.
West, J. B. (1977) *Respiratory Pathophysiology: the essentials*. Williams & Wilkins, Baltimore.
   Helpful companion to book on respiratory physiology.
West, J. B. (1979) *Respiratory Physiology: the essentials*, 2nd edn. Williams & Wilkins, Baltimore.
   Concise and readable.

1 Symptoms and signs of respiratory disease

Buller, A. J. and Dornhorst, A. C. (1956) The physics of some pulmonary signs. *Lancet* **2**, 649–651.
Forgacs, P. (1978) *Lung Sounds*. Ballière Tindall, London.

Porter, R. (Ed.) (1970) *Breathing: Herring-Breuer Centenary Symposium.* Churchill, London.
  Contains some relevant papers on the symptoms of breathlessness.

2   Basics of lung disease. Pulmonary function testing

Cotes, J. E. (1975) *Lung Function: assessment and application in medicine*, 3rd edn. Blackwell Scientific, Oxford.
Pride, N. (1971) The assessment of airflow obstruction. Role of measurements of airways resistance and tests of forced expiration. *British Journal of Diseases of the Chest* **65**, 135–169.

3   Airways obstruction

Clark, T. J. H. and Godfrey, S. (1977) *Asthma*. Chapman & Hall, London.
Fletcher, C., Peto, R., Tinker, C. and Speizer, F. E. (1976) *The Natural History of Chronic Bronchitis and Emphysema*. Oxford University Press, Oxford.
Holland, W. W. and Gilderdale, S. (1981) Epidemiology of chronic bronchitis. Chapter 3 in: *Scientific Foundations of Respiratory Medicine*. Ed. by J. G. Scadding, G. Cumming and W. M. Thurlbeck. Heineman Medical, London.
  Epidemiology review.
Thurlbeck, W. M. (1976) *Chronic Airflow Obstruction in Lung Disease.* W. B. Saunders, London.
  Review of pathology.

4   Disease of the lung parenchyma

Hunninghake, G. W. and Fauci, A. S. (1979) Pulmonary involvement in the collagen vascular diseases. *American Review of Respiratory Disease* **119**, 471–503.
Morgan, W. K. C. and Seaton, A. (1975) *Occupational Lung Diseases.* W. B. Saunders, Philadelphia.
Scadding, J. G. (1967) *Sarcoidosis.* Eyre & Spottiswoode, London.
Turner-Warwick, M. (1978) *Immunology of the Lung.* Edward Arnold, London.

5   Respiratory failure

Campbell, E. J. M. (1965) Respiratory failure. *British Medical Journal* **1**, 1451–1460.
  Key reference from which most modern thinking derives.
Sykes, M. K., NcNicol, M. W. and Campbell, E. J. M. (1976) *Respiratory Failure*, 2nd edn. Blackwell Scientific, Oxford.

Domiciliary oxygen

Medical Research Council Working Party (1981) Longterm domiciliary oxygen therapy in chronic hypoxic cor pulmonale complicating chronic bronchitis and emphysema. *Lancet* **1**, 681–686.

Nocturnal Oxygen Therapy Trial Group (1980) Continuous nocturnal oxygen therapy on hypoxaemic chronic obstructive lung disease. A clinical trial. *Annals of Internal Medicine* **93**, 391–398.

6 The pulmonary circulation

Fishman, A. P. and Hecht, H. H. (1969) *The Pulmonary Circulation and Interstitial Space.* University Chicago Press, Chicago.

Harris, P. and Heath, D. (1978) *The Human Pulmonary Circulation.* Churchill Livingstone, Edinburgh and London.

Hughes, J. M. B., Glazier, J. B., Maloney, J. E. and West, J. B. (1968) Effect of lung volumes on the distribution of pulmonary blood flow in man. *Respiratory Physiology* **4**, 58–72.

West, J. B. (1979) Blood flow. Chapter 4 in: *Respiratory Physiology: the essentials.* Williams & Wilkins, Baltimore.

West, J. B., Dollery, C. T. and Naimark, A. (1964). Distribution of blood flow in isolated lung; relation to vascular and alveolar pressures. *Journal of Applied Physiology* **19**, 713–724.

7 Respiratory infections

Cameron, I. R. and Phillips, I. (1980) Pneumonia. Chapter 9 in: *Recent Advances in Respiratory Medicine—2.* Ed. by D. C. Flenley. Churchill Livingstone, Edinburgh.

Crofton, J. and Douglas, A. (1981) Upper respiratory tract infections *and* Pneumonia. Chapters 8 and 9 in: *Respiratory Diseases*, 3rd edn. Blackwell Scientific, Oxford.

Flenley, D. C. (1981) Pneumonia. Chapter 8 in: *Respiratory Medicine.* Ballière Tindall, London.

8 Acid-base disorders

Davenport, J. W. (1974) *ABC of Acid–Base Chemistry*, 6th edn. University of Chicago Press, Chicago.

The in vivo v. in vitro controversy

Brackett, N. C. Jr, Cohen, J. J. and Schwartz, W. B. (1965) Carbon dioxide titration curve of normal man: effect of increasing degrees of acute hypercapnia on acid–base equilibrium. *New England Journal of Medicine* **272**, 6–12.
  The *in vivo* case.

Robin, E. D., Bromberg, P. A. and Tushan, F. S. (1969) Carbon dioxide in body fluids (Editorial). *New England Journal of Medicine* **280**, 162–164.
  The *in vivo* case in perspective.

Siggaard-Andersen, O. (1963) The acid–base status of the blood. *Scandinavian Journal of Clinical and Laboratory Investigation* **15**, Supplement 70.
  The *in vitro* case.

Stern, L. I. and Simmons, D. H. (1969) Estimation of non-respiratory acid-base abnormalities. *Journal of Applied Physiology* **27**, 21-24.
Some differences using the *in vivo* and *in vitro* approaches.

9 Pulmonary tuberculosis

Caplin, M. (1980) *The Tuberculin Test in Clinical Practice.* Ballière Tindall, London.
Crofton, J. and Douglas, A. (1981) Chapters 12-17 in: *Respiratory Diseases*, 3rd edn. Blackwell Scientific, Oxford.
Fox, W. (1980) Short course chemotherapy for tuberculosis. Chapter 12 in: *Recent Advances in Respiratory Medicine—2.* Ed. by D. C. Flenley. Churchill Livingstone, Edinburgh.

10 Carcinoma of the bronchus

Crofton, J. and Douglas, A. (1981) Lung cancer. Chapter 34 in: *Respiratory Diseases*, 3rd edn. Blackwell Scientific, Oxford.
Doll, R. and Peto, R. (1976) Mortality in relation to smoking: 20 years' observations on male British doctors. *British Medical Journal* **2**, 1525-1536.
Dunnill, M. S. (1982) Carcinoma of the bronchus and lung. Chapter 15 in: *Pulmonary Pathology* Churchill Livingstone, Edinburgh.
Geddes, D. M. (1979) The natural history of lung cancer: a review based on rates of tumour growth. *British Journal of Diseases of the Chest* **73**, 1-17.
Gray, N. and Hill, D. (1980) Can we stop people smoking? Chapter 15 in: *Recent Advances in Respiratory Medicine—2.* Ed. by D. C. Flenley. Churchill Livingstone, Edinburgh.
Sudlow, M. F. (1980) The treatment of lung cancer. Chapter 8 in: *Recent Advances in Respiratory Medicine—2.* Ed. by D. C. Flenley. Churchill Livingstone, Edinburgh.

Index